# How to Handle
# Your Hormones

# How to Handle Your Hormones

The essential survival guide for women of all ages

# Dr Ginni Mansberg

NEW
HOLLAND

# Contents

# A Note of Thanks

There are some people I would like to pay tribute to for giving so generously of their time, and expertise in helping me write this book; first to Daniel, my husband. I cannot ever thank you enough.

Thanks, too, in no particular order to Drs Mark Beale, Nikki Goldstein, Vincent Giampapa, Alan Kaye, David Rosen, Rod Baber, Warren Kidson and Steve Thornley. And to lifestyle experts, Ginette Lenham and Rachel Livingstone. Your generosity is much appreciated.

# Introduction

Hormones are the most life giving and vital chemicals in our bodies. We despise, vilify and misunderstand them. Being 'hormonal' may mean being moody and irrational while simultaneously being female. To many women, being 'hormonal' means crying in sad movies, eating family-size bars of chocolate for no good reason, screaming at our kids and feeling nauseous at the thought of having sex. We blame our hormones for our cravings, our bad dreams and our fatigue.

There is much misinformation about hormones. As a GP and a woman I am asked all the time to help my patients who are feeling 'hormonal'. I'm often asked for 'hormone tests'. Yet, I believe that many of the complaints that my patients think are 'hormonal' symptoms are mental health issues. Without a doubt, in some women, hormones make existing moodiness and tiredness worse though they aren't necessarily the cause. For these 'hormonal' women, often no hormone test or hormone treatment will get them back on track.

My obsession with hormones began a few years back. In 2008, I returned to full-time medical practice after taking a year out to focus on health policy in federal politics. I decided not to return to my old stomping ground in the red light area of the city where I'd spent years dealing with drug and alcohol abuse. Instead, I found my way to a new practice in the suburbs, and became one of only two women GPs there. Naturally, I ended up seeing a lot of women, many of whom complained of being 'hormonal'.

What I found among my patients was a series of serious hormonal issues that were flying below the radar and piqued my interest. The first one was hormonal weight gain. There were lots and lots of women who came to me complaining that they were struggling with their weight while swearing on a stack of bibles as high as you like that they were 'being good'. They would ask why the numbers on the scales wouldn't budge when they were following the whatever amazing, hyped-up commercial-magazine-touted diet to the letter, or spending a fortune on personal trainers and dieticians. Could they all be having sneaky chocolate bars at 2 am?

What I did notice was that many of these women had previously been diagnosed with a condition called polycystic ovarian syndrome (PCOS). I'm going to spend lots of time discussing this condition throughout the book, but in a nutshell, it's lots of cysts on the ovaries, which disrupt the normal hormonal cycle making it irregular and sometimes causing pain, infertility and acne. As you can imagine, with any condition that leaves girls never knowing when their next period is coming, many end up taking the contraceptive pill to regulate their cycle. Many of the women who had started the pill for their polycystic ovaries were convinced it was the culprit behind their battles with their weight. At the time I dismissed these women, telling them that the pill wasn't to blame. After all, that was what the text books tell us! But I wondered, could there be a connection between the irregular periods and acne of polycystic and their weight issues?

My moment of revelation arrived thanks to my (now) great friend and nutritionist, Susie Burrell. Susie had worked with hormone specialist, endocrinologist Dr Warren Kidson, for years. It was she who revealed the link between weight and PCOS and confirmed that difficulty in shifting weight IS a symptom of polycystic ovarian syndrome. I couldn't believe it. I called her straightaway and asked if she would explain the link to me in physiological terms. Susie explained the missing link was a condition called insulin resistance (IR). People with insulin resistance have too much insulin, only it doesn't work well, making the body's ability to process carbohydrates work at half speed at best. Insulin is a fat storage hormone and high insulin levels make it difficult to burn fat – hence it causes classic hormonal weight gain. It is STRONGLY linked to polycystic ovaries, the two conditions often going hand in hand. I read, searched and researched. There was so much new knowledge available since I had left medical school when PCOS was a stand-alone condition linked to infertility, menstrual cycle problems and hairiness. I discovered that there was a link, too, between polycystic ovaries and fatigue and mood problems. Exactly what most of these patients were complaining about. Wow! They weren't imagining it!

You know what it's like when you come across something that profound? I started noticing women in my practice with what I suspected was PCOS and IR and, after chatting with them about their problems, and with their permission, started ordering tests for them. The tests included blood insulin, glucose tolerance tests and androgen (male hormone) studies. Sure enough, I found this problem is common...and so misunderstood.

These were women with major hormone issues. Their hormones made life hell for them and yet, until now, what is a true medical problem had been dismissed as a lack of self control. They had spent their lives dieting and exercising and then given up in a blaze of guilt and despair. They had often consulted hypnotists, naturopaths and psychologists to help them. Often they were battling mood swings and depression as well. These women weren't suffering adrenal fatigue. No supplement would make a jot of difference. Yet medicine was failing them. OK, that was step one on my hormone obsession journey....

The second hormone problem that captured my attention in my practice materialised at around the same time. I guess like most young people I never really thought too hard about menopause. I knew that people going through the menopause have hot flashes and mood swings, but I didn't really think about how it all worked or what caused these symptoms. Suddenly, I saw patient after patient in their mid to late 40s with issues: bleeding going haywire, exhaustion, painful boobs and pelvic area, moodiness and insomnia seemingly out of nowhere. What was going on? These women clearly weren't menopausal because they were bleeding.

How wrong was every bit of my understanding of the female reproductive life? I now know that hormonal imbalances towards the end of the reproductive era mirror those that many of us had as young teens when our periods were so horrific that we had to call our mums to come and collect us from school and we had our jumpers tied around our waists to hide an unexpected flood, and we were crying from pain. The problems these women complained of were caused by an oestrogen, progesterone (and sometimes androgen) imbalance that starts as soon as the ovaries start planning their retirement.

There are so many hormone problems like those that I have addressed in this book. Fixing hormonal imbalances requires specific treatments as well as general health measures, good information and lots of understanding.

In writing this book I hope to reach out to women whose hormones might be at the root of problems ranging from mood swings to weight gain, wrinkles to low libido, fatigue and exhaustion to constipation. I discuss hormonal problems suffered by every age from teens to the menopause and beyond, and explain scientific, evidence-based information that offers a way through the hormonal mire. There is hope.

Now all that's left to say is keep reading. To the women out there trying to work out what the hell is happening with their hormones, or whether what they have could be hormonal, for the brave women who shut up and grin and bear it, this is for you. Meeting and treating all of you as your GP is an absolute privilege.

# The Hormone Primer

In this chapter I will explain what hormones are, how they work and what's happening to your hormones in certain circumstances (such as going on the pill, feeling stressed etc).

This chapter is for people who CARE about the HOW and WHY of things. If you understand something you're more likely to feel engaged and empowered. But if your heart is sinking at the thought of having to return to high school-type learning, feel free to skip this chapter altogether and get to the nuts and bolts of handling your hormones.

For those who are still with me, let's go! Strap on your thick black glasses, tuck your shirt into your high-waisted pants and let's channel our inner science nerds together. (I'll make it easy to understand... promise!!)

## What is a hormone?

Your hormones are your chemical worker bees that are products of your endocrine system. This system is spread all over the body and in simple terms harnesses the hormones it has created to control the way organs and systems in our bodies behave. Glands produce and release hormones into the bloodstream. From here they travel throughout the body finding cells that bear a specific hormone receptor on their outer cell membrane. The receptor is a chemical badge displayed somewhere on the cell, which is pur- pose- built to recognize a specific hormone. Each hormone has its own receptor, which will only become activated by its chosen hormone. The cells bearing the specific receptors are known as target cells and can be very far away from the original endocrine organ.

On reaching the target cells the hormones activate these re- ceptors chemically. If there is no receptor, the hormone will whizz past in the bloodstream without affecting the cells. Once activat- ed, the chemically-altered hormone receptor initiates a series of biochemical reactions within the cell that make the cell respond. That response might be, for example, making a particular pro- tein or changing the shape and structure of the cell. If you want to find out the detailed biochemistry of these interactions, jump on the net – I will lose 99 percent of you if I even try to go there! The reaction changes the way our body responds and makes us feel. For example, the hormone adrenaline, made by the adre- nal gland, once in the bloodstream flows a reasonable distance from some of the heart's muscle cells. The adrenaline receptors on the heart muscle cell walls detect their chosen hormone and activate, and as a result the heart speeds up and pumps harder.

There are basically two broad types of hormones:
* Protein hormones (these form the bulk of our hormones). These can't penetrate the cells. All of their actions come from activating the receptors on the outside of the cell wall.
* Steroid hormones, on the other hand can penetrate the cell's membrane and bind to the receptors located inside the cell.

Hormone receptors are located everywhere and provide a clue to exactly what the hormones do. For example, oestrogen, our favourite girly hormone, doesn't just have receptors in the female reproductive organs but in the skin and in the emotional centres of the brain as well. I know none of you will be surprised to hear that.

The reason why we are all so different and why some of us are more 'hormonal' or more susceptible to the effects of our hormones than others is because we all have different clusters of receptors on different cells and some of our receptors are more sensitive to 'normal' hormone levels than others. The site, number and sensitivity of our hormone receptors is determined by our genes.

If you have a ton of oestrogen and progesterone receptors on your brain, or they are exquisitely sensitive receptors because that's how you've been genetically predetermined, your girly hormone levels will have far more impact on your mood, your memory and the way your brain functions than women with a different brain-hormone-receptor configuration. It also explains why not everyone experiences PMS, menopause, or thyroid problems in the same way.

## The hypothalamus and the pituitary – a beautiful dance

The hypothalamus is a hormone-producing part of the brain and considered by some to be the hormone powerhouse of the body. It sits in the centre of the brain close to the point from where the spinal cord starts to take nerves out to the body. Most of its hormones it produces only need to travel a very short distance to the tiny pituitary gland buried deep in the brain.

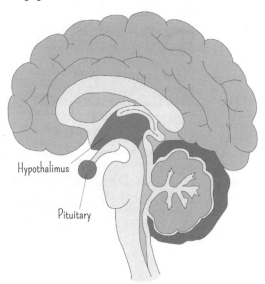

Hypothalimus

Pituitary

The hypothalamus is packed with nerves or neurons that are specialized 'neurosecretory' neurons. These function as both nerves and mini glands that secrete hormones. These secreted hormones control the release of the really powerful hormones from the anterior pituitary, a gland nestled deep in the brain. The hypothalamus is packed with nerves or neurons that are specialized 'neurosecretory' neurons. These function as both nerves and mini glands that secrete hormones. These secreted hormones control the release of the really powerful hormones from the anterior pituitary, a gland nestled deep in the brain. The hypothalamus provides an extra layer of control to ensure the system performs seamlessly. The hypothalamic hormones are referred to as releasing hormones and inhibiting hormones, reflecting their influence on anterior pituitary hormones. The pituitary itself produces the hormones that control everything from your hormonal cycle to your kidneys, adrenal glands and your thyroid. This is an action packed hormonal area.

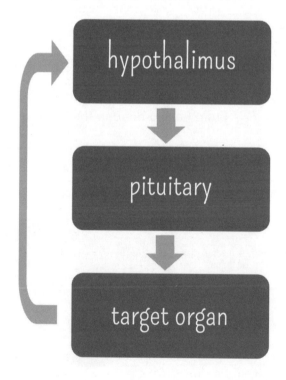

Nearly all are controlled with what we call a feedback loop. The hypothalamus releases hormones when it detects a need and switches off when the need is sated. For example, the hypothalamus will release a hormone to tell the pituitary to release another hormone to switch on the thyroid gland. When enough thyroid hormone is detected by the neurons of the hypothalamus as the blood flows through it, it arrests the GO signal to the pituitary, which in turns takes its foot off the thyroid accelerator and the thyroid gets a slow down message. In that way your hormones are always kept in fine balance with changes effective by the minute.

## Hypothalamic hormones

Let's run QUICKLY through them:

TRH (THYROTROPIN-RELEASING HORMONE)
Thyrotropin-releasing hormone tells the pituitary to switch on thyrotropin, which in turn, switches on your thyroid gland. Just to confuse things more, thyrotropin is also called TSH or Thyroid-stimulating Hormone.

GHRH: GROWTH HORMONE-RELEASING HORMONE
This hormone tells the pituitary to secrete growth hormone. See below.

GnRH: GONADOTROPIN-RELEASING HORMONE
This hormone activates the menstrual cycle in women. It all starts here.

CRH: CORTICOTROPIN-RELEASING HORMONE
In response to stress this hormone stimulates the pituitary to release corticotrophin, which acts on the adrenal glands – see below.

SOMATOSTATIN OR GROWTH HORMONE-INHIBITING HORMONE
This hormone tells the pituitary to stop making growth hormone. This hormone one is made by other tissues and not just the hypothalamus. Its focus is carbohydrate metabolism (see below) and is concerned with ensuring stable sugar levels.

# Anterior pituitary hormones

The pituitary gland is buried deep in the brain and it punches way above its weight in terms of what it does for such a tiny gland.

The posterior pituitary makes two hormones:

### ADH: Anti-diuretic Hormone or Vasopressin

This hormone kicks in especially when you're asleep and travels to the kidney to make it conserve water (make less pee).

### Oxytocin

This hormone makes the uterus contract after you've given birth. It also stimulates milk production and acts on the brain as a love and bonding hormone. Studies have shown that breast-feeding mums, with plenty of oxytocin in their bloodstream are calmer in the face of psycho-social stress than bottle feeding mothers. In a study at Bar-Ilan University, Israel, researchers found that the higher the oxytocin levels were in the blood in the first trimester of pregnancy, the better the mums bonded with their babies after birth. Additionally, the higher the oxytocin levels throughout the pregnancy and in the first month after the birth, the more likely the women were to do maternal things such as singing special songs to their little one or bathe and feed their babies in specific ways. Further research has shown that oxytocin is released in response to nipple stimulation and during (or after orgasm – it can be hard to be specific in these scientific studies!).

Oxytocin became known as the love hormone because research shows that it evokes feelings of contentment, calmness and security around a mate and lowers anxiety levels. After a positive social interaction a blood oxytocins spike can occur. But more recent research shows a less clear cut role for oxytocins. For example, we now know that oxytocin levels are high under stressful conditions, such as social isolation, being apart from a partner, or when you are sticking around in a miserable relationship along with the cortisol levels that you would expect. For more on the classic stress hormone, cortisol, keep reading. Scientists have proposed that by putting out lots of oxytocin, the brain may be trying to calm itself down and help itself through a hard patch.

The anterior pituitary makes the rest of the pituitary hormones:

### LH AND FSH: LUTEINIZING HORMONE AND FOLLICLE-STIMULATING HORMONE

These kick start the reproductive cycle (more on this below).

### TSH: THYROID-STIMULATING HORMONE

This stimulates the thyroid gland in the neck to make and release more thyroid hormone. If there was a problem in your pituitary and it didn't release enough TSH, your thyroid would go to sleep and your metabolism would be a bit stuffed given that your thyroid controls your metabolism (for more on this keep reading)

### GH: GROWTH HORMONE

Growth Hormone stimulates growth by switching on production of chemicals called somatostedins by the liver and kidneys, which, in turn make the bones grow. Growth hormone is also important for metabolism, stimulating the body, especially the muscles, to build protein. Meanwhile, it encourages the body to break down fat. Finally, it blocks entry of sugar into the fat cells so the fat cells have to eat their own fat for fuel. Studies have shown that adults get a little peak in blood levels of GH about 70 minutes after they have fallen asleep, when its job seems to be maintenance of the hippocampus. GH helps the brain process memories and solve problems while you sleep. In both human and animal studies, growth-hormone deficiency stops the brain performing as well as it might otherwise especially in complex intellectual challenges. GH also plays a role in metabolizing some of the stored nutrients during night time, when at least in theory, you should be fasting.

### ACTH: CORTICOTROPHIN (ALSO KNOWN AS ADRENOCORTICOTROPIC HORMONE)

ACTH travels to the adrenal glands sitting on top of the kidneys and instructs them to pump out the hormone cortisol. Cortisol is often referred to as the stress hormone and is pumped out in RESPONSE to perceived stress. It is an indirect measure of stress in the body rather than the cause of stress.

### PRL: PROLACTIN

PRL is best known for making the female breast produce milk. During pregnancy, prolactin levels increase by 10 to 20 times their usual level and continue at those levels if you breast-feed your baby. Interestingly, prolactin receptors are also found on lots of immune cells and it's also thought to be an immune booster. PRL stops ovulation occurring by inhibiting the body's ability to make oestrogen. It's an interesting one because it isn't stimulated by the hypothalamus; it's inhibited by the feel good neurotransmitter dopamine.

The pituitary is so busy; it's amazing more things don't go wrong with this system. (Actually things do go wrong; it's just that we never know.)

## Hormones of the pancreas

The pancreas is like two endocrine glands fused together. Most of the pancreas is devoted to the production and release of the vital digestive enzymes that are released directly into the small intestine to digest food via a duct that exists purely for this purpose. But scattered through this enzyme-making pancreas gland are hundreds of thousands of clusters of cells, which make the major carbohydrate-metabolizing hormones insulin and glucagon, plus a few other hormones.

Insulin and glucagon are the chief regulators of blood glucose levels. Sugar levels are vital. All cells use glucose as their preferred fuel. But the brain is utterly dependent on glucose as its fuel, because brain cells, known as neurons cannot use non-sugar fuels such as fatty acids or amino acids from proteins to function. When sugar levels drop, you will feel light headed, irritable, feint, possibly headachy, and unable to concentrate.

### Insulin

This is a hormone that many women come to hate. Insulin is responsible for allowing glucose, the main sugar, which serves as the cell's principle fuel, into the cells. Glucose cannot get into the heart of the cell unless insulin unlocks the door of the cell. Think about insulin as the key and the insulin receptors as the locks on the doors of the cells. This tiny little molecule is secreted by the pancreas beta cells when it senses that your blood-sugar levels have gone up or when indicated by nerves that are stimulated by the sight and taste of food.

Insulin doesn't just allow sugar into the cells, however. Think of it as the triage officer more or less in charge of how your food-based fuel gets dealt with. The presence of higher levels of insulin in the blood tells your body that it is a time of plenty (insulin is only released from the pancreas in response to the presence of food). Thus, it tells your body to start storing fuel for future periods of starvation. Instead of being expended, excess sugars are turned into glycogen, the liver's main storage form of sugar. Once the liver's glycogen storage is full to capacity, insulin instructs the liver to make fat out of the incoming sugars. These fatty acids are sent out into the bloodstream to be stored in offsite storage facilities (like your butt, thighs and round your middle). The insulin itself unlocks all the fat cells to the fatty acids sent out by the liver as well as any sugar molecules that the fat cells can use to make their own fat for storage. The last thing insulin does is to turn off fat burning. If you are like me, the thought of insulin coursing through your body turning your lithe frame into a massive fat arse is infuriating. Insulin is not your friend unless you're starving or look like a supermodel.

But wait! There's more! The last thing you would need in a time of plenty is to feel too full to eat. Insulin to the rescue! It presses its own little over-ride switch in your brain, switching off the 'I'm full' signals and tricking you into feeling hungry. People with higher insulin levels (see Are My Hormones Making Me Fat?) feel hungrier, crave more sweets, enjoy sweet things more and... no surprise, eat more than people with lower insulin levels. How annoying!

## GLUCAGON

Glucagon is the yang to insulin's yin. It raises your blood sugar levels in response to detecting a lack of glucose. Once in the bloodstream, it gets to work undoing all insulin's hard work. In the liver it instructs glycogen to release sugar into the bloodstream. Then it tells the liver to convert its protein to sugar (a simple chemical reaction). If this is not enough to raise sugar levels in the body, it instructs the body's fat cells to release their precious stored energy and convert the stored energy to sugar.

There are two other major triggers that cause glucagon to be released besides a low sugar level in the body. The first is a high level of amino acids in the blood. Amino acids are the building

blocks of proteins. This is partly why having lots of protein in your diet helps you lose weight by boosting your glucagon levels. The second glucagon trigger is exercise.

No surprises that high sugar levels in the blood switch glucagon off. So any high-sugar diet will send insulin levels soaring and glucagon levels plummeting. Guess what advice I'm going to give you in the Chapter Are My Hormones Making Me Fat?

While we're talking about hormones that control weight, the most logical next step is to discuss the rest of the metabolic hormones in the family;

## Gastrointestinal hormones

Digestion and metabolism are controlled by hormones. Most of these hormones are actually made within the gastrointestinal system and control everything from how hungry you are to how efficient your metabolism is.

### GASTRIN
This hormone is released by the stomach in response to the presence of protein. It makes your stomach pump out acid, which helps your enzymes break down the protein.

### CHOLECYSTOKININ
Made by the small intestine in response to fat inside the gastrointestinal tract. It makes the gall bladder release bile to help break down fats and tells the pancreas to release enzymes for digestion.

### SECRETIN
This intestinal hormone is concerned with acid and base balance within the gastrointestinal tract and beyond, using bicarbonate and water to keep the pH at the right spot.

### GHRELIN
This is a hunger turbo-charger. Levels of ghrelin in the blood rise just before eating and when fasting. Huge blood ghrelin level drops are noted after a gastric-bypass operation and this is thought to play a role in the weight-loss success of that dramatic

procedure. When injected into humans in a science laboratory, the food intake goes up by close to a third. Eating turns ghrelin production off, but some foods are better at switching it off than others. Meals loaded with carbohydrates and proteins dampen ghrelin release, much more than fats. Made by both the stomach and small intestine, it is also made in small amounts by the kidneys, hypothalamus, pancreas, and placenta in pregnant women. There are many ghrelin receptors in the appetite area of the hypothalamus as well as the areas of the hippocampus associated with reward. They're often switched on by drugs and other pleasurable stimuli. Ghrelin switches on growth hormone but it also ironically switches off fat burning.

MOTILIN
This hormone is secreted by the small intestines and used to make the intestine move food as well as the normal between-meal secretions that build up, for cleaning and maintenance of the guts.

# The Incretin hormones

There are two incretin hormones: glucose-dependent insulinotropic polypeptide (GIP) and glucagon-like peptide-1 (GLP-1)

Both are made in the intestine and are released in response to you eating. They help to control your sugar levels. It's important to understand these two hormones as they're at the forefront of new diabetes' treatments.

Both are fairly similar in the way they work but it is GLP-1 that interests scientists the most. GLP-1 streamlines the process of insulin release from the pancreas in response to food. It ensures a good insulin response, but makes sure the insulin is released in response to food only, instead of being constantly thrown into the blood for no good reason at all (which is what happens in Type II Diabetes). More importantly GLP-1 slows down food passing through the guts, meaning there's a slower release of nutrients into the bloodstream and making you feel fuller. GLP-1 only lasts in your blood a few minutes before it's broken down by an enzyme called DPP-4. DPP-4 inhibitors are newish drugs that help manage Type II Diabetes and help with weight loss in diabetics as well.

# Hormones made by your fat cells

### LEPTIN

This is a fascinating hormone covered in detail later, see Are My Hormones Making Me Fat? It has two key functions that make it of interest to those of us carrying more weight than we'd like and to drug companies hoping to come up with an anti-obesity drug. Firstly, it works on the hypothalamus in the brain and tells it that you're full. It also increases the sensitivity of the cells to insulin, which means that you need less of the fat-promoting insulin to get sugar into the cells. That's another boon for weight watchers. Lastly, it seems to encourage the breakdown of the storage form of fat into the more usable fatty acids.

### ADIPONECTIN

Our understanding of Adiponectin is basic, but what we do know is that it's made by fat cells and increases our body's sensitivity to insulin. It tells the body to break down fat into free fatty acids. It is a powerful natural anti-inflammatory hormone. Studies suggest that Adiponectin release can be triggered by short bursts of intense exercise. A couple of studies have also suggested that a small amount of alcohol each night can raise your Adiponectin levels and increase your sensitivity to insulin. So a red wine a night may help weight loss a little.

### THYROID HORMONE

The thyroid gland sits at the bottom of the neck, just in front of your throat. Its hormone, known as thyroid hormone, affects every aspect of metabolism. Receptors are located in almost every tissue type and the thyroid hormone determines how and what they metabolize.

Thyroid hormone is made using iodine. Without enough iodine from the diet (which is more common than you might think) the body wouldn't be able to make enough thyroid hormone. The thyroid gland makes Thyroxine AKA T4. It's not particularly metabolically active. It's more metabolically active partner is triiodothyronine, AKA T3. T3 is made directly by the thyroid in small amounts but most of it comes from the breakdown of T4 in the body, especially in the liver and kidneys. About 99 per cent of the thyroid hormone travels through the bloodstream hooked onto a protein called thyroid-binding globulin (TBG). Only the thyroid hormones NOT tied to the thyroid-binding globulin can activate the cells. The thyroid hormones hooked up to proteins just form a good reserve pool and can jump off their carrier proteins any time when needed.

Thyroid hormone gets fat to be released from its various storage sites into the blood, but on the flip side stimulates the breakdown of fats in the body for energy use. It does the same with carbohydrates. More sugars are released into the blood but the actions of insulin are sharpened meaning more sugar moves into the cells.

* Thyroid hormone hastens the passage of food through the entire gastro-intestinal tract.
* All this metabolic activity emits heat. So the thyroid hormone keeps you warm (people with an underactive thyroid can't stand the cold!)
* The thyroid hormone stimulates growth and development of all tissues in the body.
* The thyroid hormone stimulates metabolism by increasing the heart rate and the force of the heart's contractions.
* Naturally, the thyroid gland deteriorates a little with age. Levels gradually fall, although they are likely to remain in the 'normal' range.

PARATHYROID HORMONE

This is secreted by the parathyroid glands, which are tiny little cell clusters buried deep in the thyroid gland. Its principal role is to regulate the blood's calcium levels, moving the calcium out of the bones to boost blood levels. Parathyroid hormone also tells the kidneys to release calcium.

MELATONIN - THE DRACULA HORMONE

Making exclusive night-time appearances, melatonin is one of the brain's inbuilt tranquilizers. Secreted from the tiny pineal gland buried in the brain, it is triggered by darkness and switched off by light. When bright light hits the eyes, nerves in the retina at the back of the eye start firing. They are connected through nerve pathways to the hypothalamus. Within the hypothalamus, these nerve pathways activate the supra-chiasmatic nucleus (SCN), a specialized group of cells. As a result of the SCN's activities, the body's temperature starts rising, and stimulating hormones such as cortisol are released. The SCN switches off melatonin release from the pineal gland.

Usually the pineal gland starts pumping out melatonin at around 9 pm. Melatonin levels stay elevated in the blood for about 12 hours until daylight at around 9 am the following day activates the SCN, which signals the pineal gland to shut down melatonin release. During the daytime blood levels of melatonin are negligible.

Melatonin levels are affected by age. Children usually secrete more melatonin than adults, and the older you become, the less melatonin your pineal gland seems to produce. It's more complex than a simple linear relationship with age as research shows that older people with insomnia don't necessarily have lower melatonin levels in their blood than good sleepers of the same age.

Research has focused on melatonin's role as an antioxidant and immune-system booster as well.

# Adrenal hormones

The adrenal glands can be divided into two parts:

The adrenal medulla: makes the classic stress hormones, adrenaline and nor-adrenaline. These are protein hormones.

The adrenal cortex: makes three types of hormones: the so-called mineralocorticoids, such as aldosterone, which regulate your fluid, chemistry and salt levels; glucocorticoids (95 per cent of which come from the 'stress hormone', cortisol); and adrenal androgens or sex hormones. The main one of these is called dehydroepiandrosterone (DHEA). All adrenal cortical hormones are steroid compounds derived from cholesterol.

# Medullary hormones

### ADRENALINE AND NOR-ADRENALINE

Adrenaline and nor-adrenaline are made in what we call the adrenal medulla in the middle of the gland and it is completely separate from the rest of the adrenal gland. Adrenaline and nor-adrenaline are made and released into the bloodstream after direct stimulation by the local sympathetic nerves. No controlling hormone is required and it's not on a feedback loop. These are your classic stress hormones and an immediate response of your body to a perceived threat. They are responsible for preparing your body to thwart danger. They are the flag bearers of the sympathetic nervous system, the famous 'fight or flight' response. They prepare your body to outrun a predator and outfight an enemy in your midst. For all those hard and fast physical tasks you need your muscles, your brain, your eyes all to be functioning at peak performance.

Adrenaline and nor-adrenaline boost the performance of the heart by making it beat both faster and harder. It makes the walls in the arteries and veins tighten and stiffen in order to elevate blood pressure – a bonus if you're bleeding and need to conserve vital blood pressure to make sure you're getting enough oxygen to vital organs such as the brain. Together they help you get more oxygen to your muscles and brain by opening up the airways to allow the lungs to take up more oxygen. They also tell the body to start breaking down fat for usable energy and breaking down the storage form of glucose, again for easy use by the muscles and brain.

## Cortical hormones

### CORTISOL

Cortisol is a stress hormone that plays a major role in glucose metabolism and in the body's response to stress. How much cortisol your adrenal glands make is almost entirely controlled by the secretion of ACTH (Adrenocorticotropic hormone) by the anterior pituitary gland. Usually, the whole system has its own circadian rhythm, peaking in the early morning and dropping off in the evening so you can get some sleep.

Lots of minor stressors will prompt your body to release extra cortisol. Physical stresses such as sickness, fasting, exercising or simply waking in the morning, as well as psychosocial and emotional stress will prompt the body to release cortisol. Similarly, we see higher blood cortisol levels in people with medical problems such as high blood pressure, high cholesterol and pre-diabetes. It's this minor stress on the body that prompts cortisol to flow.

Cortisol has many effects on the body:

* It instructs the liver to start making glycogen, the storage form of sugar. It tells the liver and other cells to go easy on the sugar consumption. The overall result is an increase in your blood sugar levels and more glycogen storage in the liver.
* Meanwhile cortisol starts depleting the body's protein stores, stopping the body from creating new protein by getting the muscles to break down protein and release the amino acids that result into the bloodstream.
* Cortisol also affects fat metabolism. It taps into the body's fat stores (in the form of triglycerides), moving it around the body, delivering it to hungry tissues such as working muscle and to the abdomen for storage away from the storage areas under the skin around your butt and thighs.
* Cortisol is a major natural anti-inflammatory. It has a number of biochemical methods of stopping inflammation.
* While cortisol decreases inflammation, on the flip side it dampens immunity, by promoting shrinkage of the immune-generating lymphoid tissue.
* Cortisol is a weight-gain hormone. Animal and human studies have shown that cortisol injections boost appetite, creating cravings for sugar and fatty foods, which make you gain weight. There are lots of cortisol receptors in the hypothalamus that control taste and cravings. It's probably why, when you're stressed, you crave chocolate.

## ALDOSTERONE

The prime role of this hormone is balancing the sodium and potassium in the bloodstream. When this hormone is released the kidneys are instructed to deliver more potassium into the urine but to extract more sodium.

It takes on a similar role in the sweat glands, bowels and salivary glands, telling them to conserve sodium and changing the chemical composition of the fluids released. Aldosterone is also involved in a major blood-pressure hormone stimulating another cascade of blood pressure raising hormones.

ADRENAL ANDROGENS (MALE SEX HORMONES)

Some women are surprised to hear that we have lots of male hormones in our bodies. Women's levels are just five to 10 per cent of the level that men have. Androgens, including the most important and metabolically-active androgen, testosterone, are important in women's health. If there is too much or too little of them they can cause health issues. Roughly half of the male sex hormones in the body are made by the ovaries and the rest by the adrenal glands. The adrenal glands make a pool of male sex steroids, all of which can be converted into other hormones and some of which are active themselves.

Actions of androgens in women:

*   Increase oil (or sebum) production on the skin and hair. If produced to excess you will have oily skin and acne.
*   Increases the production of that wiry, coarse pubic and underarm "terminal" hair. Excess testosterone in women can be responsible for hair in unwanted places, including on your legs, the snail trail from the belly button to the pubic region, around the nipples and on the chin and upper lip. Some women have those thick coarse hairs in other places such as the chest, tummy, lower back, neck and cheeks.
*   Androgens increase hair loss from the scalp, especially the top of the head
*   They are involved in the maturing of the sex organs.
*   They increase libido and the degree of sexual arousal.
*   They increases muscle mass.
*   They increases bone density and the maturation of bone cells.
*   They increase water and sodium reabsorption from the kidneys thus increasing blood pressure.
*   They increase attention, memory, and spatial ability.
*   Testosterone is a steroid hormone, and most of that which is in the bloodstream is transported attached to a carrier protein called sex hormone-binding globulin (SHBG).
*   High androgen levels are seen in women with polycystic ovary syndrome. This condition affects your weight, looks and mood.
*   Low androgen levels are rarer and can be caused by a

whole range of problems; some medications will cause it, as will problems of the pituitary failing to stimulate the adrenal glands and ovaries to make enough androgen.

You'll notice, I didn't mention the menopause as a cause of low androgens. As you age, you might think that your androgen levels would fall along with oestrogen and progesterone, but that's not always the case. We are all so different. Some women's androgen levels drop significantly, though many women's ovaries retain the ability to make androgen for years after the menopause despite the fact that the ovaries are no longer able to produce oestrogen and progesterone. Relatively, these women will have more androgens than oestrogen as they age so they develop a hormone imbalance with hairs on the chin, fat around their middles and hair loss on top of the head.

Regardless, in ALL women (and men for that matter) testosterone can be converted back to oestrogen by an enzyme called aromatase that is present in the ovaries and the fat cells. As we get fatter, we make more aromatase, which means we lose more androgens in favour of oestrogen. Testosterone levels vary in all women as they age, with some women maintaining good levels, some having them drop off and others having too much.

### DHEA

DHEA (dehydroepiandrosterone) hormones are a big pool of highly flexible sex hormones that can easily be converted to either oestrogen or testosterone in the tissues. They do nothing themselves, and you should view them as a useful mob of pre-hormones that the body converts into whatever it feels it needs. We start producing DHEA at around six to eight years of age. Blood levels of DHEA peak between the age of 20 and 30 years and after that they slowly and steadily decline. By the time you are 70 years of age, your blood levels of DHEA are 10–20 per cent of their peak levels.

Studies have shown that if you have blood levels of DHEA below the 10th centile (the lowest tenth in terms of sheer numbers), you have a greater chance of having sexual problems such as low libido or difficulty reaching climax, both before and after you start menopause. Other studies have linked low blood levels of DHEA with a lower general feeling of wellbeing in women. Certainly anti-ageing specialists, especially in the USA, believe that taking a DHEA supplement may have anti-ageing effects. It's a popular hormonal therapy for that reason but it's never taken off in the mainstream medical world because the science is lacking. The quality of the trials has been too poor to conclude much and for every positive result there's a negative one to counteract it.

Stress and chronic illness, both of which dampen your libido also suppress your DHEA levels. It may be that low DHEA doesn't cause the sexual problems, but rather both low DHEA and low libido are symptoms of stress so treating one will at best only give you a placebo effect. See Are My Hormones Destroying My Sex Life?

### PREGNENOLONE

Apart from its role as a precursor to DHEA, pregnenolone also directly stimulates the brain. This hormone inhibits the neurotransmitter, GABA, which is your brain's built-in sedative, reducing excessive brain activity and promoting a state of calm. Research is underway as to whether pregnenolone could be used to counteract age-related memory loss and poorer brain function. There have been conflicting results from studies, though plenty of people report feeling sharper while taking it.

### ALLOPREGNANOLONE

This hormone switches on our GABA receptors and has both sedative and anti-anxiety properties. It is a product of progesterone from the ovaries and is independently made by the adrenal glands. The adrenals seem to pump out allopregnanolone along with all the fight and flight hormones in response to stress to keep us calm.

Recent studies of returned servicemen from Iraq and Afghanistan in the US found that the lower the allopregnanolone levels in the blood, the higher the chances of post-traumatic stress disorder. A good response to treatment saw allopregnanolone levels increase.

### ANDROSTENEDIONE

This is another reserve hormone, which is a precursor to oestrogen and testosterone. It is made by a chemical reaction altering DHEA. There are two sources of androstenedione in the body; the first is in the adrenal gland, like DHEA. The rest is made by the ovary (or testis in men). In the ovaries, luteinizing hormone stimulates the thecal cells that line the outside of the stimulated ovarian follicle to make androstenedione. This is then converted to oestrogen and progesterone within the ovary.

In the uterus, a baby's androstenedione levels slowly increase, peaking at birth. Levels fall dramatically during your little one's first year of life and stay very low, rising again in the lead up to puberty and reaching adult levels around age 18. The source of the increase is the maturing adrenal glands. Levels start to fall and by menopause they're very low again.

Now let's get to the nitty gritty of hormone world. These names are going to run through the rest of the book, so let's get familiar with the main players in a girl's world:

### OESTROGEN

The word oestrogen really refers to a group of hormones; Oestrone (E1), Oestradiol (E2), and Oestriol (E3) plus 50 lesser known hormones. Oestradiol is the most common, the strongest and the most well studied of the oestrogens. Oestrone is weaker than oestradiol and is the more common oestrogen seen in post-menopausal women, and oestriol is the weakest oestrogen of all and is a major player during pregnancy. The body can easily switch one hormone into any of the other oestrogens at any time. Oestrogen hormones are all made in the ovaries out of cholesterol but small amounts are also made from adrenal sex hormones and fat cells.

Oestrogen has a number of roles, mostly sex related.
* It is the major player at puberty, without it a women wouldn't develop breasts or pubic hair.
* It also controls the menstrual cycle. Under oestrogen's steady influence, the uterus grows stronger; the vagina walls become thicker and more moist.
* Oestrogen stimulates the brain, which can be great for thinking and memory, but at its extremes can make you

feel anxious, agitated and even cause migraines and fits.

* It instructs your liver to make more HDL, the good choles-terol and less LDL, the bad cholesterol.
* It can control where in your body you store your fat. Your fat cells also have oestrogen receptors and oestrogen tells your body to deposit more fat in the girly spots on the thighs and butt and on the breast and less on the tummy.
* The skin has oestrogen receptors and becomes plumper when there's more oestrogen.
* There are oestrogen receptors on the bone cells. Oestrogen stops bone loss, keeping bones strong.
* Oestrogen increase the body's ability to make blood clots.
* In the gastrointestinal tract, oestrogen slows down the bowel's movements but increases production of bile from the gall bladder.
* It encourages the kidney to retain fluid and salt.
* It improves the health and tone of the entire urinary tract, helping defend against urinary tract infections.
* It boosts production of sex hormone-binding globulin (SHBG), a protein that binds androgens in the blood-stream making them less active.

Just take a look at this extensive list. It seems that cells in al-most every system have oestrogen receptors and are affected by our menstrual cycle and our hormones.

As you age, less oestrogen comes from the ovaries and more comes from other sources. The first of the non-ovarian sources is the, albeit shrinking pool of adrenal androgen precursors. The second and equally important source of post-ovarian oestro-gen comes from an enzyme we met in the section on androgens called aromatase, which sits in both your ovaries and your fat cells and converts testosterone to oestrogens.

PROGESTERONE

I thought I would start here by clearing up some of the nomencla-ture around progesterone. All progesterone comes under an um-brella term of progestogens. They're the steroid hormones that act like progesterone (see below). When we say 'progesterone', it refers specifically to the natural progestogen you make in your

33

ovaries. Progestins are artificial progestogens we give you in tablet or other form to help with hormonal issues or for contraception. OK? Let's continue....

Progesterone is the other significant female hormone, produced by the ovaries. It is made by the corpus luteum, which is made up from the leftover cells of the ovarian follicle after it has released its precious egg into the fallopian tube to be fertilized. If you are pregnant, progestogens are also pumped out by the placenta. The role of progesterone is to help you get and stay pregnant. A small amount of progestogen is also made from the adrenal glands via conversion from pregnenolone.

Progesterone receptors are found all over the body, but being a steroid hormone, the receptors are located within the cells. Let's look at some of its actions:

* Progesterone makes the endometrium more habitable for an embryo, but also makes it more compact and less likely to grow out of control.
* Progesterone thickens the cervical mucus, making it thick and impenetrable to sperm.
* It is a natural nerve cell calmer, calming and even sedating on the brain. Progesterone helps you sleep properly
* It makes you more likely to burn fat as an energy source.
* It makes you hungry.
* It is an anti-inflammatory hormone and dampens down your immune system's ability to respond to a bug, etc
* Progesterone plays a role in increasing your thyroid hormone levels.
* Progesterone has a role in controlling blood sugar, copper and zinc levels.
* It has a diuretic effect on the kidneys encouraging them to release more salt and water, in effect countering the action of oestrogen.
* It also counters oestrogen's shove along to the body's clot-making system. Progesterone basically makes clotting LESS likely.
* Progesterone allows the muscles that line the walls of the arteries and veins to relax, making blood pressure fall and sometimes contributes to swelling in the hands and feet in pregnancy or the second half of your menstrual cycle.

* Progesterone is amplified by oestrogen, which increases the number of progesterone receptors in a cell when it is around. In return, progesterone makes the oestrogen receptors function more effectively, making them more sensitive to smaller amounts of oestrogen.

# The 'normal' menstrual cycle

To understand what can go wrong with your hormones, you need to understand what happens when everything works well. For this explanation I'm going to assume that your cycle is 28 days. Of course, the reality is that many of us have cycles that are longer or shorter than 28 days. Bear with me as it's just easier to explain it this way.

Girls are born with about two million ovarian follicles. Of these, only about 400 will mature enough to be able to ovulate during your child-bearing years. The rate at which you lose those follicles over time is mostly a result of your genes.

In a miraculous process, one follicle is selected each month, often from alternating ovaries, to become mature and release an ovum or egg. We are not entirely sure how that follicle is selected but we do know that the follicles are priming themselves to get their cues to start turning into mature follicles around five months before it actually happens. During this time the cell structure of the immature follicle starts to change and it grows more of a cell known as a granulosa cell, in effect a hormone-producing factory.

This process, known as 'pre-follicular development' is continuously happening so your ovaries have follicles of varying stages of maturity all the time.

## Days 1–5 (your period)

Let's call this the baseline with all hormone levels at zero. Low levels of the main female hormones, especially progesterone allow the hypothalamus buried deep in your brain to pump out GnRH (gonadotrophin-releasing hormone). With lots of GnRH pumping around, the pituitary gland releases the first important hormone of your cycle; follicle-stimulating hormone (FSH). Once in the bloodstream, the FSH travels down to your ovaries. When it rises to a specific level, it stimulates the pre-primed follicle that sits in the ovaries to start developing and maturing. The follicles have two important cells that start making hormones:

* Theca cells lining the outside of the follicle, which start pumping out androstenedione.
* Granulosa cells in the centre of the follicle, which convert the androstenedione to oestrogen. The granulosa cells also provide nutrient-rich fluid to bathe the unfertilized eggs which are growing in the core of these follicles.

## Days 6–10 (early pre-ovulatory phase)

The mature follicle starts to grow more FSH receptors, which means that there is more FSH around, and that the follicle is responding to it. Under this heavy influence of FSH, the primed follicle with theca and granulosa cells working beautifully together pumps out oestrogen in the first half of the cycle causing a little peak of oestrogen without progesterone in the first half of the cycle. In the first half of the cycle oestrogen is in a dominant phase. In one to two per cent of cycles your ovaries mature two follicles equally, which increases the possibility of twins, although that is more likely to happen as you get older.

The build-up of oestrogen in the blood has a couple of effects. Firstly, it works on the endometrium (lining of the uterus), thickening the nutrient-rich blood for any potential embryo to bury into and feed from. This is called the follicular endometrium. In the ovarian follicle, in response to the increasing FSH and oestrogen, the follicle's granulosa cells grow luteinizing hormone (LH) receptors on their surface.

## Days 10–13 (late pre-ovulatory phase)

The second effect is the higher levels of oestrogen feedback to the hypothalamus, which then stops releasing as much GnRH and as a result switches off the pituitary's production of FSH so levels of FSH start to drop off.

# Day 14 (ovulation)

Unlike FSH, in response to the rising levels, the pituitary releases LH in a surge causing fluid to flow into the follicle, making it swell to 0.5–2 centimetres. The LH makes the walls of the follicle thin and brittle so that they break down easily and release their egg. The ligaments between the ovary and fallopian tube contract, pulling the ovary closer to the fallopian tube, allowing the egg, once released, to find its way into the tube. The egg release happens between 16 and 24 hours of the LH surge. The whole ovulation process takes two or three minutes. The release of the egg isn't necessarily automatic. The follicle must have grown and be mature enough to be able to be stimulated by the LH. Mucus in the vagina also thins to allow sperm easier access to the cervix and the available egg.

# Days 15–22 (luteal phase)

The remains of the follicle minus the released egg becomes known as the corpus luteum. The corpus luteum releases masses of progesterone along with tiny amounts of oestrogen, pregnenolone and androstenedione. The luteal phase of the cycle is progesterone-dominant. The luteal phase of the cycle is progesterone-dominant. Progesterone is responsible for making the uterus favourable for a new embryo. It takes the oestrogen-readied endometrium and basically perfects the formula. It organizes the blood vessels and provides enough glycogen for the hungry embryo to feed on. Progesterone also travels though the bloodstream back to the hypothalamus in the brain and tells it to switch off the GnRH tap, ensuring that levels of FSH return to zero.

One other hormone produced by this corpus luteum is inhibin, which switches off any response to FSH and makes sure no other follicles start developing too soon.

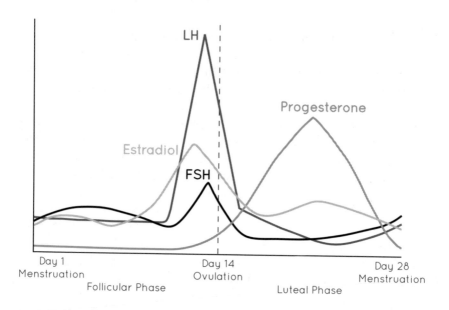

## Days 23–28

Assuming fertilization hasn't occurred, the corpus luteum fades away (now called the corpus albicans) and stops producing oestrogen and progesterone. The drop in oestrogen in particular means that the endometrium starts shearing off the wall of the uterus and you get a period.

Eventually blood levels of this hormone fall low enough to stimulate the hypothalamus to start pumping out GnRH again and the cycle starts again.

## What happens to your hormones when you take the contraceptive pill?

This cycle doesn't happen.

Broadly speaking, there are two types of hormonal contraceptives, combined oral contraceptives and progesterone only contraceptives. With combination contraceptives both oestrogen and progesterone are used, while with 'progesterone'-only formulations... you guessed it... we just use progestins.

Let's start with combination contraceptive pills, the ones that are more common and that you can assume people are talking about when they discuss 'the pill'.

When taking the combined contraceptive pill oestrogen is at relatively high levels in your blood and the hypothalamus is not triggered to produce GnRH. As a result, your pituitary will not produce FSH and your ovaries will not start to prepare a follicle in the ovaries. No follicle means no egg. You read that correctly, women on the pill do not ovulate. This means you won't have an egg waiting to be fertilized by sperm should they come swimming around looking for a party. That party is already significantly shut down; the progesterone makes the mucus in the cervix much thicker and less penetrable by sperm anyway.

If you add up the total monthly amounts of oestrogen and progesterone in your blood, they are roughly the same for women on the pill as women who aren't on the pill. It's just that oral contraceptives create an even blood level throughout the cycle and even out the spikes and dips in the hormone levels that are seen as part of the routine cycle. So, being on the pill won't make you more 'hormonal'. In many ways you become less 'hormonal' because your hormone levels remain stable. Many of the symptoms of PMS (see Are My Hormones Making Me Moody?) can be mitigated by the pill by simply ironing out the peaks and troughs in your hormone levels.

## 'The pill', the combined oral contraception (using oestrogen and progesterone)

The standard pill has two hormones in a single tablet. Both oestrogen and progestogen are included and have a dual action to stop you getting pregnant. The oestrogen in the pill negatively feeds back to the hypothalamus telling it there is plenty of oestrogen on board, just like a pregnancy. This effectively tricks it into not releasing any GnRH. As a result the pituitary doesn't produce any FSH and voilà, the ovary doesn't get triggered to start producing an egg. It really is that simple. You won't ovulate and if an egg is not released from your ovaries, you can't get pregnant. As a back-up, the pill also does all the things that the progesterone-only contraceptives do (more on this below), such as thickening your cervical mucus making it impenetrable to sperm.

## PERIODS ON THE PILL

The reason you have 'periods' on the pill is largely historical. When the pill was being developed, the makers thought that women would not cope well without having something resembling a normal 'cycle'. How would she be able to tell if she were pregnant, for example? So the pill makers designed the pill to be split between 21 days of active pills (pills containing oestrogen and progesterone) and a pill-free seven day 'period' (where you either take no pills or sugar pills). The rapid fall off in oestrogen levels creates an oestrogen 'withdrawal bleed', which looks very similar to a period.

You don't need a period of course. It doesn't cleanse or detox you. Contrary to the misogynistic view of menstrual blood as dirty and a way of releasing female angst or whatever other rubbish is out there, a bleed is something to make women feel like they're having a normal cycle even when they're on the pill. From my perspective, you're better off without them. You don't need to lose blood and precious iron each month (see Are My Hormones Making Me Tired?).

You also don't need to lower your oestrogen levels to the point where you risk a pregnancy. You see, with this break of seven days, you are bordering on ovulating. If you forget to go back on hormone tablets and start your new pill packet late, chances are you will ovulate and if you have unprotected sex, you may get pregnant. And how easy is it to start a pill packet late? It's so easy to forget to restart, especially if you're not in the habit of actually taking your sugar pills. It's the same issue if you miss the last few active pills before the sugar pills. Whether it's by forgetting to take them, or whether it's because you go on antibiotics or have some vomiting or diarrhoea, missing pills near your sugar pills puts you at risk for pregnancy.

Lots of girls remember from a normal cycle that you can't get pregnant during your period. At that time you have no endometrium and the egg has fallen over, but you haven't started making a new egg yet. So it's confusing that your 'period' on the pill is your MOST fertile time because you're not protected by the hormones.

For that reason I always recommend 'tricycling'. No, not on the trike you rode at pre-school! Tricycling on the pill means taking three active packets together without a pill -free or sugar pill 'period' so, in effect, you have four 'periods' a year instead of 12. Some women get breakthrough bleeding doing it this way. It doesn't mean you'll get pregnant but it does mean you'll be annoyed! If that happens, you can try 'bicycling'. You guessed it; that means taking two active pill packets back to back and skipping every second period.

Another advantage of skipping 'periods' on the pill is the steady hormone levels. If you suffer from headaches, mood swings and other issues from the fluctuations in your hormone levels (see Are My Hormones Making Me Moody?), either off the pill or on a standard pill that causes your hormone levels to drop off a cliff every four weeks, this could really help you. You can get some breakthrough bleeding in the first few months, but usually it goes away if you push on with it. There are now more and more pill regimens that allow you to skip periods altogether. Chat to your GP if you are really sensitive to the effects of your hormones and having a steady level throughout the year sounds like a good option to you.

### MISSING A PILL

So by now you've probably worked out that missing a pill in the middle of the pack is the safest time to do it because you've got a good buffer on each side. Just take it when you remember it and keep going. If you miss three or more pills, you will bleed, but you can keep taking the pills anyway. You'd be unlucky to ovulate after only three days off the pill but it has been known to happen so most doctors suggest using condoms just in case.

### TYPES OF COMBINATION PILLS

There are so many and deciding which is right for you can be difficult. Broadly speaking there are monophasic and multiphasic pills. In monophasic pills, which are the most common, the active pills are the same dose every day. In multiphasic pills, the amount of hormone in each one varies, so you can't substitute days and you can't really bicycle or tricycle.

Then there are the Rolls Royce pills and what I call the Camry pills – you know, good, reliable, nothing flash, gets you from A to B. No extra special features. I'm a fan of Camry pills unless there's a specific need you have to address a hormonal issue.

The listed advantages and disadvantages of each type of pill are based on clinical studies. So, let's go through some of the pills on the market:

### STANDARD PILLS (CAMRYS)

**Contain:** 30–35 micrograms (mcg) of Ethinyl Oestradiol plus progestin (the types of progestins vary between brands, which are either norethisterone or levonorgestrel).

Norethisterone is the so-called first generation progestin. Levonorgestrel is a second generation progestin. The second generations have a higher androgenic effect than the first generations – although both have much higher androgen effects than third generations or anti-androgen pills (see below). The androgen effects come from being metabolized by the liver into some testosterone. That's why they can make some women break out in zits and raise levels of your bad cholesterol. I'm a big fan of Norethisterone and will tend to pull that out as my first line pill (as most of my patients will tell you) but many docs love the second generation progestins and at the end of the day, in 90 per cent of women it won't make much of a difference.

**Examples:** Microgynon30, Nordette, Levlen, Monofeme (all with levonorgestrel) and Norimin, Brevinor (Norethisterone). All are monophasic.

**Advantages:** Cheap, you can get a year-long prescription, reliable work horses.

**Disadvantages:** Some women will be hit hard by the androgen effects. It's not common but some will get acne and hair loss on the head because so much of the progesterone gets broken down to testosterone. They just have to switch pills to a Rolls Royce.

### ANTI-ANDROGEN (MALE HORMONE) PILLS

**Contain:** 30–35 mcg of Ethinyl Oestradiol plus progestin with anti-androgen properties called Cyproterone Acetate. Cyproterone acetate is a progestogen derivative that blocks the androgen receptors making testosterone's effects remarkably less noticeable.

**Examples:** Diane-35, Brenda, Estelle and Valette. All are Monophasic

**Advantages:** These pills are designed to combat an androgen build up if you have that happening. They are absolutely fantastic for women with excessive hair growth (on the body or face), acne, hair loss (from the head) because of excess androgens, especially from Polycystic Ovarian Syndrome (PCOS) (see Are My Hormones Making Me Fat?). The beneficial effects on the greasiness of the skin happen within weeks although the full effects on your acne and excess body hair might take a few months to kick in. Wonderful, wonderful when you have too much androgen in your body.

**Disadvantages:** They're Rolls Royce pills so yes, they are much more expensive and can reduce your libido, especially if you didn't have excess androgens in the first place. Only use these if you have a specific reason to do so. Anti-androgen pills have been delisted in France because of their increased risk of clotting. They are being investigated in other countries.

### Low dose pills

**Contain:** 20 mcg of Ethinyl Oestradiol plus progestogen.

**Examples:** Microgynon20, Loette, Microlevlen. All are monophasic

**Advantages**: The low oestrogen dose is really good if you get nauseous, or have breast tenderness, bloating and headaches on the higher dose of the pill.

**Disadvantages:** There is a higher risk of breakthrough bleeding with the lower dose pills. They're also more expensive than Camry pills.

### Multiphasic pills

**Contain:** Each of these pills is slightly different, but will have between 20 and 40 mcg of Ethinyl Oestradiol progestogen. The pills change as you advance through your cycle.

**Examples:** Trifeme, Triphasil, Triquilar, Logynon. Multiphasic so the amounts of Ethinyl Oestradiol and progestin vary throughout the course of the cycle.

**Advantages**: They're designed to mimic a natural cycle

**Disadvantages:** Where do I start? Firstly, missing a couple of pills can be really confusing. Then the fluctuating hormone levels mean these pills give some women mood swings. Plus there's a possibility of an increased breast cancer risk (still to be confirmed). I just don't use them at all.

### Third generation pills
**Contain:** 30 mcg of Ethinyl Oestradiol and specialized third generation progestin such as gestodene and desogestrel.
**Examples:** Marvelon, Minulet, Femoden. All are monophasic pills.
**Advantages:** The third generation progestins are less androgenic (less prone to breaking down into testosterone) and also don't have any of the mild oestrogen effects of the Camry pills. As a result, they've been linked to less weight gain and less acne.
**Disadvantages:** Studies have linked third generation progestins to a slightly higher risk of blood clots compared to classic progestins. They're also more expensive.

### Fourth generation pills
**Contain:** Either 20 mcg (Yaz) or 30 mcg (Yasmin) Ethinyl Oestradiol and Drospirenone, a fourth generation progestin. It is said to be closer to your natural progesterone. It is made from a diuretic called spironolactone instead of testosterone. It is also a mild anti-androgen, blocking testosterone from activating its receptors. It is as effective as the Cyproterone acetate containing pills for acne.
**Examples:** Yaz and Yasmin. Both are monophasic pills but Yaz has 24 active and four inactive (sugar) pills. Yasmin has the usual 21 active and seven inactive pills.
**Advantages:** It's all about the progestin. We have good evidence that pills containing Drospirenone can really help with the symptoms of mild PMS, such as increased appetite, moodiness and fluid retention (see Are My Hormones Making Me Moody?). It's also a great choice for acne. The combined mood and acne effects have made these the most popular pills in the USA.
**Disadvantages:** Women who take contraceptive pills containing Drospirenone have a six- to sevenfold risk of developing potentially fatal blood clots compared to women who aren't on the pill, and a twofold risk compared to women who take a pill with a different progestin. Having said that, the total risk is still low. It's also super expensive. Because it also counteracts the actions of Aldosterone

(see above,) you can end up with too much potassium in your system. That's so rare, I don't really see it but if you have an issue with your kidneys, your liver or your adrenal glands, steer clear. Your GP wouldn't prescribe it for you in that case anyway.

# Progesterone – only forms of contraception

Lower dose progesterone-only contraceptives, such as the 'mini-pill' can sometimes stop you ovulating, but you shouldn't count on that. They mainly work by thickening the cervical mucus, making it impenetrable to sperm.

High-dose progestin-only contraceptives, such as the injectables Depo-Provera or Depo-Ralovera actually do stop you ovulating as well as having the same cervical mucus changes as the low dose progestogens.

### THE MINI-PILL
**Contain:** 30 mcg levonorgestrel (progestogen) or 350 mcg norethisterone (progestogen).
**Examples:** Microlut, Noriday.
**How to take it:** You take the same pill every day, within a set three-hour window otherwise it won't work. If you're even an hour late, you have to use other forms of contraception for two weeks. So work out whether you're a morning or evening person and make sure you're always close to your pill at that time.
**Advantages:** If you're breast-feeding, it won't interfere with your milk supply. It is also an option for women who cannot take any oestrogen because they have had breast cancer or have very high blood pressure or smoke and can't take the risk of blood clots (see below).
**Disadvantages:** You get a very narrow window (three hours) to take it each day. So if you take the mini pill at 8 am, and you haven't taken it by 10 am you can't rely on it as a contraceptive and have to use something else (withdrawal, condom or abstinence). Plus it's not as effective a contraception as a combination pill. In the ideal world, if you take it at the same time every day, you only have a 0.3 per cent chance of becoming pregnant on the mini-pill. In the real world, where the pill gets taken late or forgotten altogether, eight per cent of women can expect a pregnancy each year.

### PROGESTOGEN IMPLANTS

**Contain:** Etonogestrel as an implantable rod that is put under the skin of your arm and slowly releases progesterone over three years.

**Examples:** Implanon, Nexplanon.

**Advantages:** Set and forget. It eliminates the possibility of mistakes, such as forgetting a pill or two leading to pregnancy. It is fully reversible. If you have it taken out, you're back to normal in no time. It's cheap. It lasts for three years so is much more cost-effective than getting a monthly pill prescription.

**Disadvantages:** It has to be inserted by a doctor who has done some special training. Not all GPs do it (I don't). Some studies suggest there is a tiny increased risk of breast cancer for up to 10 years after use of the rod. Ditto cervical cancer.

### PROGESTOGEN-RELEASING IUD

**Contain:** Levonorgestrel is contained within the IUD and around 20 mcg per day is released (compared to about 30 mcg on the mini-pill). The dose is so low that 85 per cent of women continue to ovulate on the Mirena.

**Examples:** Mirena.

**Advantages:** Again, it's set and forget. It eliminates the possibility of mistakes, such as forgetting a pill or two leading to pregnancy. It is fully reversible. If you have it taken out, you're back to normal in no time. It's cheap. It lasts for five years so is much more cost effective than a monthly pill prescription. A BIG advantage is that the progestin is released directly into the uterus, thinning the lining and making your periods really light – we're talking panty liner for a couple of days light. As a result, it's a brilliant option for women with heavy periods from any cause (once it's been investigated by your doctor of course!).

**Disadvantages:** It has to be inserted by a doctor who has done some special training. Not all GPs do it (I don't). It is inserted via a speculum and some women find that insertion process uncomfortable. I've used them since the birth of my last child and don't find it a problem. There have been reports of more acne and breast tenderness with them. See *Are My Hormones Making Me Look Bad?* and *Are My Hormones Destroying My Sex Life?* for more information.

# The pill and cancer

I thought I'd put this in here because it is something so many of my patients ask me about. In 1996 the Collaborative Group on Hormonal Factors in Breast Cancer did some analysis of more than 50 studies worldwide and found that women who were either on the pill or had recently stopped did have a very slightly higher risk of breast cancer than women who had never used the pill. The earlier you started taking the pill, the higher the risk, the researchers said. They also found that once you'd been off the pill for 10 or more years, the risk of breast cancer returned to normal baseline levels.

More recently than that the latest results from the enormous, ongoing Nurses' Health Study, which has been following more than 116,000 female nurses (24 to 43 years old at the start of the study in 1989), confirmed the link between being on the pill and a very slight increase in the odds of getting breast cancer. But in this study, further analysis showed that the increased risk, as small as it was, was seen almost exclusively among women on 'triphasic' pills, (like Triphasil) where the dose of hormones changes in three stages over the month.

Meanwhile, almost every study has found that being on the pill lowers the risk of ovarian cancer. Back in 1992 a huge analysis of 20 studies revealed that the longer you've been on the pill, the lower your risk of ovarian cancer. For example, the risk went down by 10 to 12 per cent after a single year of taking the pill and down by 50 per cent after five years of pill use.

Similarly, all studies show a decreased risk of endometrial cancer when the pill is taken, and as with ovarian cancer, the longer you take it, the lower your risk.

Studies have found that being on the pill increases your risk of cervical cancer. But before you panic, experts don't think the pill is to blame. It may just be that if you're on the pill, you're more likely to be sexually active and you have less need for condoms. Given that most cases of cervical cancer come from contracting a sexually transmitted infection, the link might be a coincidence.

# Peri-menopause

There comes a time when your ageing ovaries can't go through the same cycle any more. They simply can't go on cyclically producing hormones and releasing eggs. Ageing ovaries stop being able to respond in the same way to LH and FSH. That means your ovaries are no longer going to be able to produce oestrogen and progesterone, although other tissues can still make oestrogen.

Most women don't wake up one day with non-functioning ovaries, having had them going at full capacity the day before. Your hormone levels don't suddenly stop one day, or do they go decline evenly. Most women slowly drift into menopause, with their ovaries' production of oestrogen and progesterone becoming erratic and unpredictable at this time. The whole ovarian winding down process starts up to ten years (but typically six years) earlier than the actual menopause.

This is the most horrendous time for women. Without a doubt, it's the years leading up to that single menopausal point that give so many women hormonal grief. This starts happening from the mid to late 40s for most of us. The clues that you are approaching menopause are many but initially your periods start changing. Sometimes they become heavier and longer. Often they get more frequent. But they can get lighter from time to time and less frequent too so that you might lose track of when they're due. The peri-menopause is different for everyone. And it can be different for one woman from month to month – all depending on your hormones.

For example, if you don't ovulate one month, which becomes more common for women in their late 40s, your corpus luteum won't develop so you won't get a release of progesterone, but your oestrogen levels may continue to rise. On top of that, as you get older, your aromatase activity increases, especially if you put on weight as aromatase is activated in fat (see above). Aromatase converts your circulating testosterone to oestradiol. Your adrenal glands are already on their downward decline because of age, which has nothing to do with menopause. So you are producing less DHEA to be turned into testosterone. However, while your ovaries are not making as much girls' hormone any more, they are still quite capable of making testosterone, and the extra aromatase converts much of the circulating ovarian testosterone to oestrogen, adding to the imbalance between oestrogen and progesterone.

This has a number of effects:

* Oestrogen in the uterus unbalanced by progesterone makes your endometrium build up without packing down. As a result it is overgrown and unstable. You may have spotting all through the cycle or heavy bleeding when you do get your periods (see Are My Hormones Making Me Tired?).

* Any irregular bleeding has to be checked by a doctor. Although it's common at this peri-menopausal time, it can be a sign of something more sinister, such as cancer. Although it's rare it's a brave woman and an even braver doctor who banks on it being normal and doesn't look into it further.

* Oestrogen in the brain is not balanced by progesterone in the brain. This can give you insomnia.

* The oestrogen-progesterone imbalance together with insomnia can give you mood swings.

* The testosterone, meanwhile, can build up in some women, again not counterbalanced by oestrogen making them sprout chin hairs but lose hair on their heads.

Because of the erratic nature of your hormones at this time it can be difficult to manage the symptoms since they vary from cycle to cycle. If you are living in hormone hell, this book has some answers that may help.

# Menopause

Menopause isn't official until you haven't had a period for 12 consecutive months, and there's no other reason for that to happen (such as because of a hysterectomy). The average age of menopause is 49 or 50 (depending on the study). Early menopause is defined as occurring at any age younger than 40 and that happens in one per cent of women naturally and another six per cent of women because of surgery, or chemotherapy for cancer.

Menopause happens when your ovaries can no longer produce any oestradiol (E2). Instead, you now get most of your oestrogen by the conversion of androstenedione, from the adrenal cortex, into oestrone (E1) by peripheral tissues, and by the conversion of testosterone to oestradiol by aromatase in fat. If you remember, oestrone is eight times less potent than oestradiol.

Two thirds of women develop menopausal symptoms. The rest sail through without an issue. If you do get symptoms, this is what you may experience:

* Hot flashes (can happen at night to wake you up)
* Tiredness
* Mood swings
* Vaginal dryness
* Low libido
* Insomnia
* Less bladder control

Genes are the main determinants of your menopause, so ask your mum what happened to her. If you're a smoker, on average you will reach the menopause two years ahead of when you would have done had you been a non-smoker.

The following won't determine when you reach menopause:

* The age you were when you got your first period
* How much alcohol you drink
* How fit you are
* Your race
* Your height
* Your BMI
* The number of children you've had
* Whether you ever went on the pill

A large UK study found that having had a hysterctomy hastened menopause, probably by restricting the ovaries' blood supply. Endometriosis (a condition where the lining of the uterus doesn't stay inside the uterus but travels around the pelvis) also tends to bring on an earlier menopause.

## Diagnosing menopause

Lots of women ask me to test for 'hormones' when doing standard blood tests to diagnose menopause. Such tests are really unhelpful, especially in peri-menopause. Once you are fully though the menopause your FSH will be high and your oestrogen levels low. But in the years leading up to menopause, these tests are rarely of any use because your hormones are unreliable.

The bottom line is that you often know in retrospect that the feelings you had, the mood swings, the weight gain, the fatigue, the loss of libido were from peri-menopause.

## Menopause symptoms

Recent studies have found that the vast majority of menopause symptoms, such as hot flashes, insomnia and mood swings, last for an average of four to five years after they start but they can go on longer. By age 66, 15 per cent of women, (and 10 per cent of women over 70) still have persistent menopause symptoms. That's a whopping 10–20 years post-menopause.

One group of symptoms don't get better. They get worse. Vaginal dryness, weak pelvic floor muscles and problems with urine (leakage, frequent infections, etc) remain and often worsen with age.

# Are My Hormones Making Me Tired?

Of all the reasons that I get asked to investigate hormones, the most common is tiredness. Let's face it, lots of us are tired, especially women. We work stupid hours, women still do the bulk of that laborious, thankless, monotonous housework, we still bear the bulk of responsibility for our kids and our parents. So yes, we're tired.

But there is a difference between feeling like you could do with a week in Hawaii and feeling like you can't make it up the stairs. Or, feeling horror when you realise it's only 3 pm and you already feel like getting into bed, never mind facing another couple of hours of work, then the commute and the cooking and housework.

So let's walk through the myriad hormones that can (and do) cause exhaustion and how you can rebalance your hormones.

## Is my thyroid making me tired?

Everyone knows about the thyroid gland. Patients are often the ones who ask me to check their thyroid. The hormones the thyroid produces affect so many parts of our life; metabolism, brain development in children, body temperature, muscle strength, the dryness of our skin and hair, our menstrual cycles and our weight.

Inside the thyroid gland are lots of follicles, which vary in size. Their main job is to make the all-important thyroid hormones: T4 and, to a lesser extent, the more metabolically active T3. T3 has a much stronger effect on your cells than T4. In fact, only 20 per cent of your T3 is made in the thyroid gland. The rest is made in the body when T4 breaks down and gets rid of its central iodine molecules, converting the T4 into T3. One third of circulating T4 is converted to T3 in your tissues.

Your thyroid hormones circulate around, either joined to a protein or hanging loose and as a result, more available to hop onto the various cells in your body and activate them. T3 tends to be less tightly joined onto proteins than T4. That's the reason T3 is more powerful than T4.

But here's the important bit: the thyroid not only controls the metabolism and release of vital nutrients, it has a direct impact on the brain. We know that thyroid hormones play a critical role in the brain, dramatically having an impact upon both your mood and your brain power or 'cognition'. An under-functioning thyroid left untreated can lead to terrible depression and dementia in older adults. Without a doubt, thyroid problems definitely make you feel tired. An over- or underactive thyroid affects 10 per cent of us at any one time.

## The underactive thyroid

Altogether 80 per cent of people with thyroid problems have an underactive thyroid and most feel tired. Often they don't realise they have a medical problem. So many of my patients have put up with an under-performing thyroid for a long time by the time it is diagnosed. Often they can't believe how good they feel once they get it treated. Besides bone-weary exhaustion and weakness, people with an underactive thyroid can have weight gain from a slowed metabolism, dry hair and skin, as well as thinning hair or hair falling out. They suffer constipation; and tend to feel the cold. Swelling or puffiness of the skin can be a problem, and in women, their menstrual cycle can become very irregular.

The thyroid can be put under pressure from many causes. The main ones are Hashimoto's thyroiditis, an immune system problem where the body attacks its own gland; iodine deficiency (theoretically rare in developed countries but becoming increasingly common); and medical causes such as over-treatment for a hyperactive gland; or medications.

## The overactive thyroid

Everyone with an overactive thyroid is tired, but there are other symptoms including feeling weak, having heart palpitations, anxiety, losing weight, insomnia, tremors in the hands and diarrhoea. If you had Grave's Disease, the commonest cause of an overactive thyroid gland, you might also have puffy, dry, irritated eyes, which can sometimes bulge a bit.

The other main cause is a thyroid nodule. Nodules are actually very common, and they very rarely cause a problem but sometimes they can become overactive. We call these overactive nodules 'toxic' because they start producing masses of thyroid hormone.

## Diagnosing thyroid problems

In my experience, thyroid issues can be tricky to diagnose from a patient's history and examination. The symptoms of an underactive thyroid are so common; who isn't tired? who doesn't get constipated? (Constipation is possibly the least discussed issue in general practice but so many of my patients suffer in silence for years. Suffice it to say if I ask about bowels it seems everyone's constipated and that's not all due to thyroid issues); who doesn't get dry skin (in winter that's ubiquitous); or some ankle swelling (women with a menstrual cycle are often a bit swollen at some part of the cycle)?

So many women who are diagnosed with a thyroid issue after having a blood test are those I wouldn't have picked. Conversely a few of those patients in whom I'm convinced their thyroid glands have lost the plot have a normal test result.

To diagnose a thyroid problem, we start with a blood test. Thyroid stimulating hormone (TSH) can be measured and is a good place to start. If your TSH is high, it means it isn't being switched off because it is continuously being stimulated by a high level of TRH in the blood coming from the hypothalamus. Your hypothalamus would stop producing TRH if there was sufficient thyroid hormone about. And this would allow the TSH to fall. So you can assume that a high TSH means low thyroid hormone levels.

But that's not always the case. Sometimes the TSH level is abnormal because of a problem with the pituitary gland. The pituitary can be affected by a tumour although that is very rare.

If results of the TSH test are abnormal, one or more additional tests are needed to help determine the cause of the problem.

T4 TESTS
High T4 tells us you have an overactive thyroid gland. Low T4 tells us you have an underactive thyroid.

Sometimes total T4 levels are abnormal because the proportion of the T4 joined to a protein is not working as it should because of abnormally high or low concentrations of the protein that binds the thyroid hormones. That's why we also measure free T4. A normal free T4 level, alongside a T4 reading that is high or low, tells us there is a problem with the binding protein, not the thyroid. We see that problem in pregnancy or in women taking the pill where the oestrogen and progesterone hormones raise the levels of binding protein in the blood. In these cases we would see a high T4, and as long as the free T4 reading is low the thyroid is fine. People who use steroid medications for asthma, arthritis, or other health problems may have lower binding protein levels. Ditto other medicines for abnormal heartbeat and some other rarer medical conditions.

T3 TEST
Only about 20 per cent of the T3 in the bloodstream comes from your thyroid gland (as opposed to T4 which is made 100 per cent by the thyroid gland). If you remember, T3 is far more active than T4. It is unusual, but in some cases of an overactive thyroid, the free T4 level is normal but free T3 is raised or low. That's why doctors order it: to diagnose those rare cases.

I should just say that I often see problems with the thyroid-stimulating hormone only. Often the T4 and T3 readings are normal. That doesn't mean you don't need treatment or that you shouldn't be experiencing any symptoms. It's just that your thyroid condition is at an earlier stage and is in a milder form.

### ANTI-THYROID ANTIBODY TEST

When your immune system attacks your own thyroid gland, it does so with antibodies, which can be measured with a simple blood test. The most common culprit for an immune system attack is Hashimoto's disease.

### IMAGING TESTS

Armed with your thyroid test results we may want to investigate further. Sometimes your doctor might want to LOOK at the thyroid gland as well. Especially if the thyroid is enlarged (your doctor can usually feel it by placing fingers at the base of the throat), or if there is pain at the area of the gland or a lump. If the thyroid is enlarged a doctor may order an ultrasound scan of it. It's a simple test with no needles. A radiographer smears very cold jelly over the area, which allows a probe to move gently over your neck. The sound waves bounce off the thyroid and back onto the screen so it's possible to see whether the gland looks normal.

Other tests you may be sent for study how the thyroid gland is functioning or looking and use nuclear medicine diagnostic scans. Yes, we are talking radioactivity, but a tiny amount that won't harm you. In these scans, you swallow or are injected with some radioactive material that binds to your thyroid gland so that a special gamma camera can pick up the radioactivity inside the gland.

A biopsy is the ultimate test in which a doctor uses an ultrasound to guide a needle into the thyroid gland and take a tissue sample, which is sent to a pathologist to investigate.

What matters most of course, having got to the bottom of the diagnosis, is how to manage this hormone imbalance.

## How to handle your underactive thyroid

### MEDICATION

The best treatment for an underactive gland is to replace the missing hormone by taking a tablet every day. In most cases, we only replace the thyroxine or T4 and trust that your body will break that down to provide you with adequate amounts of the T3. Very rarely do we need to give T3 although it is available.

Getting the level right can take a few weeks, or months in the worst-case scenario. Thyroid hormone therapy fixes the problems with almost no side effects. Thyroid hormones need to be kept refrigerated and are issued with a prescription from a doctor who will monitor your TSH levels to confirm you're on the right dose. It takes a full six weeks for the blood levels of your thyroid hormone to stabilize and after that time most of my patients are feeling much better.

Your diet matters when you start thyroid replacement therapy. You need to avoid taking your thyroid hormone tablets at the same time as the following because they can make the thyroid hormone tablets less effective:

* Walnuts
* Soybean flour
* Iron supplements or multivitamins containing iron
* Calcium supplements
* Antacids
* Some medications (check with your pharmacist)

As you get older, your doctor may need to make adjustments to your thyroid replacement medication. Sometimes we lower the dose because as you get older you may become more sensitive to medications and you start metabolising and clearing the drugs in your system more slowly. You may realise your dose is too high if you feel hot or develop palpitations, or it may be picked up on a routine blood test

Many people, however, need more thyroid replacement hormone to keep their thyroid levels in balance as they age. This is because their thyroid function naturally declines over time. Once again, you might notice you feel tired or feel the cold and think immediately of your thyroid. Alternately, it may be picked up on a blood test. It does go to show the importance of monitoring your thyroid hormone levels, especially when you're on medication.

### THE THYROID HORMONE-BOOSTING DIET

Almost all of my patients ask about a diet to help their thyroid hormones and yet sadly, there is no thyroid-boosting diet. Although claims about hypothyroidism diets are rife, there's no evidence that eating or avoiding certain foods will improve thyroid function.

Having said all that, I should put in a word about iodine. When I was at university as a medical student, iodine deficiency was something that happened in the third world. In fact, we know that iodine deficiency is the most common preventable cause of mental retardation in the world. But we had plenty of iodine in our diets and it came chiefly from two sources; iodised salt and the vats that dairy farmers stored their milk in.

Today many of us use non-iodised salt and dairy farmers don't store their milk in vats that leach iodine into the milk. All of a sudden we're seeing iodine deficiency in the developed world. For pregnant women a lack of iodine in the developing baby can manifest as a lower IQ and brain issues for the baby. Pregnant women need 220 mcg per day of iodine to have enough for themselves and their baby. All pregnant and breast-feeding women should take a supplement without testing for iodine levels first.

The rest of us need 150 mcg of iodine a day from our diet. It shouldn't, in theory, be an issue, as a quarter of a teaspoon of iodised table salt provides 95 mcg of iodine, but you need to make sure your salt is iodised. Or if you like seafood, you're in luck because fish including tinned salmon and shell fish are probably the best sources of iodine. Just 170 grams of ocean fish yields 650 mcg of iodine. Seaweed is full of iodine (see table below) and so is sushi.

Below is a list of foods and their iodine content to give you an idea of how much they contain.

| FOOD | IODINE CONTENT (MCGS PER 100 G) |
| --- | --- |
| Oysters | 160 |
| Sushi (with seaweed) | 92 |
| Tinned salmon | 60 |
| Bread (baked using iodised salt) | 46 |
| Cheddar cheese | 23 |
| Eggs | 22 |
| Regular milk | 13 |
| Seaweed | Up to 4500 mcg in just 7 grams of seaweed |
| Canned tuna fish | 10 |
| Meat (beef, pork and lamb) | 1.5 |
| Tap water (varies depending on location) | 0.5–20 |

In theory you could overdose on iodine but it is rare. Symptoms of iodine poisoning include burning of the mouth and throat, fever, nausea, vomiting, diarrhoea, a weak pulse and coma. But don't worry about this. I've never seen it and you'd have to set out on a mission to overdose on it.

Selenium deficiency can also affect the thyroid. Iodine is essential for the synthesis of thyroid hormone, but selenium is essential for making the iodothyronine deiodinase enzymes that are needed for the conversion of thyroxine (T4) to triiodothyronine (T3).

We all need 55 mcg of selenium per day in our diet and the richest source is Brazil nuts. Six Brazil nuts provides 544 mcg of selenium, 85 grams of canned tuna yields 68 mcg of selenium, and 170 grams of chicken provides 48 mcg. One egg has 15 mcg and pasta also contains selenium.

### HERBS FOR THYROID PROBLEMS

The prescription of a well-regulated thyroxine hormone replacement medication is the obvious solution for me when looking at managing an underactive thyroid, but some of my patients baulk at the suggestion and want to know what herbal options they can take as an alternative, or even as an additional booster to their medication.

There are plenty of herbal and other products marketed as being able to boost thyroid function. They also claim to be safe and beneficial for general health. Recently in the USA, researchers put some of these products to the test. Of ten over-the-counter 'natural' thyroid products they found medical grade T3 in nine and thyroxine (T4) in five samples. In some of these products, taking the recommended doses, would give you T3 and/or T4 doses equal to or greater than that which a doctor would prescribe. As you'd be medicating yourself, you would have no supervision. Added to this the drugs are made without appropriate levels of safety compared to prescription drugs. Three cases of severely overactive thyroid have been reported, one of them fatal, after people took these herbal preparations. The herbal culprit contained contraband animal thyroid tissue as well as medication-grade thyroid hormones.

Some herbs that may be of interest include: *Withania somnifera* (Ashwagandha, or Indian ginseng) because it is said to have anti-ageing properties, sedative and anti-inflammatory effects, as well as boosting T4 levels. Studies in mice have shown it is a thyroid stimulant. Two other herbs, *Bauhinia purpurea* (purple orchid) tree bark extract and *Bacopa monnieri* (Indian pennywort) extract, were also found to boost both T4 and T3 levels in mice. However, we don't know what doses to use and what the long-term effects are in humans, and we don't have good human studies.

I really think that tiredness caused by thyroid hormone problems is best handled by a doctor and not a complementary therapist. The best naturopaths I know agree and I've had lots of referrals from ethical therapists who tell their patients that this problem is best handled by a medical practitioner.

## Managing the overactive thyroid

Overactive thyroid can be frustrating to manage. Often we just wait and see whether the thyroid settles down over time and even becomes inactive. This can be frustrating for the patient because they're feeling dreadful, and being told to ride it out is not great when you're trying to work and run a family. Treatment options include:

## MEDICATIONS FOR AN OVERACTIVE THYROID

Anti-thyroid drugs have been used for overactive thyroid since the 1940s. They stop the thyroid gland from making quite so much T4. It starts to work between two and eight weeks. The biggest problem with these medicines is their side effects. Allergic reactions with horrible fevers, rashes and joint pains are suffered by up to five per cent of patients, usually within the first few weeks of treatment.

Most doctors prefer to use radioactive iodine instead. A single dose of radioactive iodine is prescribed as a capsule or liquid. Because iodine is absorbed by the thyroid and no other tissue or organ in the body is capable of holding onto it, we see almost no side effects with this therapy. While we're waiting for the treatment to work, or for the thyroid to settle on its own we can use other medicines to control palpitations and hot flashes.

Only if you have a massive goitre (swelling) that is stopping you from swallowing, if you refuse radioactive iodine, or if you are pregnant and unable to wait until after the baby is born to start treatment, you may be offered the removal of the thyroid gland, although it's less common now. Removing the thyroid gland is a major operation since it contains your parathyroid glands, meaning you have an entire system to sort out afterwards. Plus, there's a chance of damaging the recurrent laryngeal nerve that controls your voice box and runs through the thyroid.

## HERBS FOR AN OVERACTIVE THYROID

If you are committed to herbal medicine, there have been studies in mice show that *Moringa oleifera* (West Indian bean leaf) extract slows down the conversion of T4 to T3 in the female (not in male mice) so there may be a potential use for an overactive thyroid gland because less T3 means less active thyroid hormone. Similarly *Aegle marmelos* (Bael tree) extract, also decreased T3 and increased T4 in a study of mice. Hardly any of these herbs have a human study to back them up and you can understand my reticence to endorse any of them. But if you want to give them a go, chat to a herbalist and discuss the potential side effects and any potential interactions with medicines you're taking first.

# Are my hormones causing my insomnia?

Are you a pillow thumper? You're in good company. We know up to 18 per cent of the population suffers from insomnia at any one time, and that these tossers and turners are approximately twice as likely to be women. The differences between men and women when it comes to insomnia become amplified as we age. By 65 years old, women are 75 per cent more likely to suffer from insomnia than men.

Any imbalance of oestrogen and progesterone can wreck your sleep. Let's have a quick re-cap of specifically how hormone imbalances can hammer your sleep:

### PROGESTERONE

We know that progesterone is a sedative hormone. If you've ever been pregnant you will remember feeling like face planting into your spaghetti bolognese, especially early in the pregnancy when progesterone levels rise at a rate of knots.

This hormonal relationship was confirmed recently when a US study established progesterone's role as a sedative by running post menopausal women (who are very low in progesterone) through a battery of tests in a sleep lab. Taking a progesterone tablet at 11 pm improved both sleep duration and sleep quality compared to a placebo. This study data is new and needs to be confirmed with larger research projects.

Studies have shown that over 50 per cent of women in the post natal period after giving birth have insomnia even when baby is managing to nap for a few hours straight during the night. That's because they've had a sudden withdrawal of progesterone, which had been high during pregnancy. After the birth you won't ovulate for a while. Even if your ovaries aren't producing oestrogen, you're still getting some oestrogen conversion from your adrenal hormones and from fat (via aromatase conversion of testosterone). So with oestrogen dominance many women will struggle to sleep.

And of course the transition through peri-menopause is a nightmare for sleep with the insomnia drama happening in as many as 50 per cent of women. Once again, you are still getting oestrogen but no progesterone because your ovulation is sporadic or your corpus luteum isn't working as well. Oestrogen switches on your brain and there's no rebalancing, calming progesterone to switch it off.

Lack of progesterone doesn't have the same effect on everyone. Some women suffer terrible insomnia in the second half of their menstrual cycle just before their period, when there's actually a dominance of progesterone. It's probably because the body temperature heats up by up to half a degree making you HOT. Heat is a sleep killer. As you will remember, your genes determine the number, placement and sensitivity of hormone receptors which is why we all have different responses to the hormones in our bodies.

If you are thinking a progesterone tablet may be a good option for your sleepless nights, there are lots of doctors using this with apparently fairly good effects. A word of warning though; progesterone does also make you hungry, so weight gain is a potential complication. But if you want to give it a go, the dose is 2.5 mg progestin. This is usually compounded into drops by a compounding pharmacist with a script from your doctor. One to two drops per night before bed. Chat to your GP about this.

### Cortisol

This stress hormone is a sleep killer. Anyone who has ever had to take 'steroid' tablets knows that as even small doses can wreak havoc with your ability to get off to sleep. Usually in your body, as the evening progresses your cortisol levels start to wane so your brain can relax and sleep. But stress states can see that cortisol natural ebb and flow through the day go pear shaped.

Sleep deprivation is a huge stressor on your body and is a good illustration of what can go wrong with cortisol. Once you have gone through sleep deprivation for more than a couple of days your evening cortisol levels go to hell in a hand basket, averaging six times the same levels of people who've been sleeping well. The high cortisol levels make it hard to fall asleep and as a result your body gets more stressed, pumps out more cortisol and so it continues. Chronic insomniacs know exactly what I'm talking about.

So whether it is your stress or your menopausal or post baby progesterone crash, your hormones can kill your sleep. And let's face it; if you can't sleep well, you're going to feel tired. So what can you do about it?

### MELATONIN

Quick recap: melatonin is the sleep hormone. A natural sedative, it runs your body clock, telling you to sleep when it's dark and to wake up when it's light. It wanes as you get older, which might be why insomnia gets more common with age. But bottom line is that melatonin is good and we want more of it!

# How to handle your insomnia

### HRT (HORMONE REPLACEMENT THERAPY)

Many of my patients are scared witless of HRT. But it is highly effective for managing the insomnia that affects half of all menopausal women. Firstly it will reduce your hot flashes making you cooler and your sleep less interrupted. Secondly, if you take combination HRT with oestrogen and progesterone, you will benefit from the sedative effects of the progesterone. Even for the most nervous Nelly, for whom the thought of HRT induces a state of panic, being sleep deprived is a nightmare for your physical and emotional health. If menopause is robbing you of your sleep, you should at least discuss this with your doctor.

Alternatively, as I said before  lots of doctors prescribe progesterone only for insomnia associated with hormonal changes.

### DIM THE LIGHTS IN THE EVENING

We're aiming to switch on your melatonin. Bright lights simply confuse your pineal gland into thinking it isn't sleep time yet and making it dull down melatonin production. Give yourself a good hour before your scheduled sleep time without light stimulation of your pineal gland for best effects. This especially works for people whose melatonin levels are somewhat awry.

### COOL IT!

As any menopausal woman can tell you, being too hot is a sleep killer. Whether it's your flannelette pyjamas, your winter weight doonas, your closed windows and absence of a fan in summer, something will have to change to get your night time temperature into a more moderate range. Now if you are one of the many women who are freezing come bed time and reflexively don your heaviest (not to mention sexiest) winter pyjamas and bed socks and huddle under the doona only to do a sweaty midnight strip tease, try these tips: Warm up before bed using a hot bath, a shower or heating, then wear light pyjamas to bed and get the right weight doona for the season. Open windows (with decent fly screens) and fan are no brainers!

### INSECTICIDE

The midnight mosquito raid is torture for poor sleepers in the summer months in hot countries. Try either putting on some insect repellent before getting into bed, or use one of those electrical mozzie repellents through the night. If you have insect screens, it is time to have them checked and repaired.

### LIGHT OUT

If you have issues with sheer curtains, raging street lights or the hall light on for tiny tots outside your door, you might find they interfere with your sleep. Try rearranging your bedroom furniture to face away from the light. And little night lights that plug into a power point do the job for little ones as well as the bright over-head variety.

### MATTRESS TIME

How old is your mattress? The mattress companies tell you to change them over every ten years. Not only do old mattresses give you uncomfortable human shaped divots in the surface that you roll into and get stuck in, but they are also full of mould and dust mite faeces that can give your allergies a good work out if you have hay fever.

### MELATONIN SUPPLEMENTS

These are available on prescription from your GP. The evidence for them working in people with jet lag and in those of us over 55 is pretty good. Taken an hour before bed time they improve your sleep and as a result your quality of life. For those of us under 55 the evidence is a little shakier. Despite that, I have had lots of patients who benefit from them. As you can't really measure melatonin levels in the blood it is hard to work out who would benefit most from them but if you are an insomniac, it would be worth a shot.

### ANTIHISTAMINES

Diphenhydramine and doxylamine are over-the-counter 'first-generation' antihistamines that have sedation as a side effect. They're also the main ingredient in a lot of the over-the-counter sleeping tablets you can get at the pharmacy. They last in your body for around nine hours so many people feel a bit woozy the next morning. Doctors have mixed feelings about them, but in my experience they work well with no addiction. Best for Friday nights or a time when an antihistamine hangover won't ruin your day!!

### LOW DOSE ANTIDEPRESSANTS

There is one called mirtazapine which has sedation as a side effect. You need a script from your GP for this one but currently it is not approved as a sleeping pill, only as an antidepressant. There are a couple of problems with it. Firstly it is approved for use as an antidepressant only so you need to understand you would be using it for a condition for which it isn't approved. Also, they can make you starving and long term, weight gain can be a problem. That puts many of my patients off!

### BE A TEETOTALLER

Sorry to be the usual party pooper but drinking to excess will destroy your sleep. Tired people often have a drink at night, especially insomniacs who are trying to medicate their way out of their chronic brain overstimulation. An American Sleep Guru, Thomas Roth said recently; "alcohol can only do one of two things to sleep: it can make it worse or it can make it much worse." As he explains, as alcohol gets metabolised, one of the by products is aldehyde and this chemical affects the brain to fragment sleep. Not immediately but as the night wears on. So you might fall asleep in a heap but you won't stay there long. If you're an insomniac, drinking makes no sense. Once your sleep is under control you can restart. In moderation of course!

### BINNING THE CIGARETTES

Smokers are worse sleepers and giving up smoking will help the quality of your sleep. A recent German study found that smokers sleep for a shorter period of time, take longer to get to sleep, have more rapid eye movement (less deep) sleep, more sleep apnoea (see below) and leg movements in their sleep than non-smokers. Giving up is a no brainer when you consider the links to blood pressure, heart disease, cancer and the cost of your fags.

Most of my patients who smoke have tried at least once to give up smoking and failed. Either they never made it through the first day or they ended up back on the cancer cigs after some reasonable period of time but circumstances conspired against them and a stressful situation put them back to square one.

So if you have tried everything, here are some thoughts that in my experience can work wonders; firstly do NOT try to give up until you're ready to hurt a BIT. That means giving up during a restructure at work or while your dad is battling terminal bowel cancer is almost set to fail. The problem with failing is that in your mind you chalk up the number of failures to mean something – although it doesn't. "I've tried a hundred times to give up – I just can't do it." Then you give yourself a legitimate excuse to fail every time and you go into each attempt not really expecting a good outcome. Without realising it you can end up sabotaging your own efforts to quit. Lots of failures simply means you had multiple errors in timing or application. It doesn't mean you are addicted for life and CAN NEVER give up. Waiting another month won't hurt (unless you're pregnant in which case, yes time is of the essence).

Then my next tip is to give up slowly if you can't go cold turkey. Let me be clear; there is no safe level of smoking. But the more you smoke, the worse for your health and on the flipside, the less you smoke the better. Most smokers tell me that not all cigarettes are equal. Some cigarettes are incredibly enjoyable and they look forward to them and enjoy them. Others simply get lit and smoked with nary a second look. So my advice is to analyse your smoking and work out which cigarettes are being smoked mindlessly then bin them.

SLEEP HYGIENE OVERHAUL

Bad sleepers often have very poorly trained brains that could use a touch of training. The idea of sleep hygiene is to clean up your bad sleep habits and retrain your brain to know when it's sleep time and when it's not.

* Wind down. You need a wind-down period before bed. This is a good hour or so to allow your overstimulated brain to wind down. No screens of any kind, be they TV, iPad, iPhone, etc. Also no heart stopping books or arguments! Instead try soft music, an aromatherapy bath, dim lights, and maybe a nice orgasm if you have a partner that is willing and able!

* Try to get to bed at around the same time each night. The idea here is to switch your body clock back on. Get your body used to associating sleep with a certain time each day.

* Step three is to train your brain to wake up roughly the same time every day, give or take half an hour. Barring an all-nighter with the toddler who has an ear infection, or other exceptional circumstances, your brain needs to learn to wake up in the morning and feel bright and awake during the daytime. This routine includes weekends. Not forever, just until we sort out your brain and get you sleeping well again.

* Bed is for sex and sleep only. There is a fallacy that 'just resting' in bed is good for your brain. But it actually has the opposite effect, making it harder for your brain to fall asleep later on and wrecking your sleep hygiene!

* Relax. Once you get into bed (or have finished having sex), practise progressive muscular relaxation in bed, in which you relax your muscles one by one from the tips of your toes to the top of your head.

* The 15 minute rule. Give yourself 15 minutes to fall asleep. If in that time your head starts to wander or you feel tense, get up and leave the room for a short time, somewhere between 10 and 30 minutes, and then return to bed as if you were starting the night again. It doesn't matter what you do as long as you don't overstimulate your brain

with a screen! You can even get some housework done. But if you're awake anyway, at least you'll achieve some productive work and not feel quite as frustrated as you would when you're just lying and watching the clock for hours at a time.

# Are teenage hormones making me (or my teen) tired?

With three teenagers at my place, I know all too well that teenagers don't like going to sleep at night. "I'm not tired" coming from a 15-year-old is different from the yawning declaration to the same effect from your four-year-old.

Two thirds of teenagers and their raging hormones have what we call 'delayed sleep phase syndrome' (DSPS). A teen with DSPS basically shifts their entire body clock backwards so that they don't fall asleep until midnight if you're lucky and two or three am if you've got a nasty case. They will then want to wake at lunch time the next day. Some of these teens (especially boys) seem to be half asleep most of the day (ask any high school teacher how common that is!) and get a burst of activity come the evening.

We know that testosterone (the male hormone) plays a role in this disorder but we're still unclear as to the exact role of the hormones. Then there's the first world issue of access to technology making the 24 hour body clock disaster easier to perpetuate.

## How to handle your (or your teenager's) insomniac hormones

Firstly, you are not going to get anywhere with any of the strategies I'm going to list below until your teen is on board. Getting your teen to buy into the need for more sleep will mean understanding what motivates them. If they're academic, they might be interested in the studies that have shown that the ideal amount of sleep for teens is 9.25 hours per night. And that getting adequate sleep is worth lots of hours of studying. If your teen is appearance conscious, it would be worth mentioning that getting enough sleep is also linked in studies to less weight gain and less pimples. If their behaviour is putting stress on their relationships, you should mention that studies have also linked getting the right amount of sleep to less depression and less anxiety. Hopefully they will get on board. The problem is that schools aren't flexible in their hours and a 6:30 am wake up is the norm for many kids. It's a dilemma for parents. If so, here's what I suggest:

### GO FOR PEACE
Make your teen's room a tranquil environment. If they have DSPS, I'd avoid self-expression in the form of black paint and heavy metal rock posters. Instead go for calming colours like pale blues and greens, cream and white.

### TECHNO CEASEFIRE
I have to admit that as a teen if I'd had access to a whole gang of buddies ready to Skype or Facebook chat to me, or posting funny memes on Instagram, I'd have found it hard to shut down my laptop. I cannot believe the number of pings from Whatsapp and sms that come in post 10 pm at night for my kids. So when you go for a techno ceasefire, you're simply going to help your teen avoid the temptation of social media and communication after 9 pm. Your teen will react with horror to the news of the new rules. Trust me. But this is going to have to be not negotiable if you are going to retrieve your level-headed, non-moody teen.

### PUSH THE SPORT
Sport is great for teens. It helps reduce anxiety and depression, prevents chronic diseases, keeps their bodies slim and zit free (they like that). Plus it will help them get to sleep a little easier.

### NO CHAOS
Get your teen organised. Get him to have his bag more or less packed and his school uniform ready to go so he can get a few extra minutes of sleep in the morning. And showering at night will help with that too.

### NANNA DINNER
Have dinner earlier if possible. Having big meals close to bedtime can keep your teen awake as digestion stimulates stomach acid, which can take an hour or more to settle down.

### Bin the energy drinks

Caffeine intolerance is very individual but lots of us get pretty geed up by caffeine. Energy drinks in the afternoon, or a latte for that matter, is asking for trouble in teens with DSPS.

### Melatonin magic

Supplementing your teen's body with melatonin is an idea that's really taken off recently even though the studies that have been done on this have yielded pretty mixed results about its efficacy. The best evidence for melatonin supplements is for short-term use. Unlike in older adults, sleep specialists suggest taking a dose of it straight after school or around six hours before bed. I have used this in my young patients with DSPS and the results have been fantastic. You will need to get prescription from your doctor for this.

# Is my menopause making me tired?

If you are in the hormone hell of peri-menopause or established in your menopause and you don't feel tired, count yourself lucky. Most women who are at this stage of life find they feel pretty flattened.

We have already established that oestrogen is a natural upper. Initially as you enter peri-menopause and your ovaries stop pumping out progesterone, sleeping and feeling calm can be elusive. Once you are fully in menopause and you're also short on oestrogen, your brain is no longer getting stimulated by the oestrogen highs. So that goes part of the way to explaining why menopause can be so exhausting for some women. But by far the biggest sleep killer for women going through menopause are hot flashes and night sweats. They're experienced by two thirds of women as they transition from peri-menopause into menopause and closer to 100 per cent of women who have an artificial menopause (for example having ovaries removed or taking some medications for breast cancer). If you're lucky you will get a flash or two every day or two and they'll only last for a few months. But lots of women can experience them ten or even twenty times a day and they can last for 15 or 20 years. Few women can stay asleep through a flash and if they come with night sweats, there can be a change of sheets on the cards! That's a lot of interrupted sleep.

We still don't know exactly what causes these two connected problems but it seems to happen when you had oestrogen in your system and then lose it. And we know putting oestrogen back into the system settles them down

# How to handle your hot flashes

### HORMONE REPLACEMENT THERAPY (HRT)

I see so many women who are simultaneously crippled by hot flashes and terrified of using HRT. So I thought I should look at the evidence with you in the hope of convincing at least some of you to go with the most effective, proven and easy way of eliminating hot flashes, HRT.

'Won't HRT give me cancer?'

In 2002 the women of the world were shocked when the huge USA based Women's Health Initiative (WHI) study was terminated early because of a 24 per cent increased risk of breast cancer in women on 'combined' HRT, a combination of oestrogen and synthetic progesterone. Subsequently, the researchers did more analysis and found that women starting HRT at least in the early stages also had a higher risk of heart disease as well.

The WHI was an impressive trial by any standards. A 15-year long study of 160,000 women, examining life and death for women once they had travelled through the menopause. The worrying statistics were confirmed when the UK based Million Women's Study (MWS) results were released in 2003 finding similar results. The media loved it. Bad headlines were ubiquitous.

Women all over the world chucked their patches and pills in the bin and decided grinning and bearing their hot flashes, their mood swings, their insomnia and aches and pains was a price they had to pay to avoid breast cancer. Doctors agreed and started advising women on HRT to get off it. So what if they'd get osteoporosis from lack of oestrogen? Today, across the world, less than 30 percent of women are getting any sort of treatment for their menopausal symptoms whatsoever. In fact so low has the demand for HRT become that lots of drug companies simply stopped making these medications and the range available to women today has shrunk dramatically. What an absolute tragedy for women.

For a start, the WHI study is deeply flawed. Let me explain why. Firstly, the average age when starting HRT in the WHI was 63 years. Think about it. For most women, by the time they're 63, their menopausal symptoms have usually finished and almost nobody in the right mind would START HRT. But it wasn't really highlighted in the reporting of the study at that time.

Here is another fact that was omitted from the reporting; the majority of subjects in the WHI were either overweight or obese, both major risk factors for breast cancer and heart disease.

Sure enough, expert groups around the world have taken great steps to assure women that this aversion to HRT has been way overblown. Ten years after the WHI results were first released, a consensus statement was put out by the North American Menopause Society, the Endocrine Society, and the American Society of Reproductive Medicine, and the statement was then endorsed by another 12 top medical societies in the USA, Canada, and Mexico. In the new statement, these major peak bodies have clearly stated that HRT is a great option for women with moderate to severe hot flashes and night sweats. They have gone as far as saying it is the best treatment available for the symptoms of menopause.

The key to successfully using HRT, they said, is to understand its limitations and how to get the best out of it. For example, HRT is best started in early menopause, in other words within 10 years of the start of menopause symptoms or by age 59. That's the sort of advice that makes sense. Hot flashes are at their worst early on in the menopause so is naturally the best time to start HRT. The next bit of advice is to use the lowest dose possible to keep the flashes under control. As they pointed out, it was the group of women on HIGHER doses of HRT that again were more likely to suffer from cancer and heart disease. Well that is easy enough to do. We start with the lowest dose and move upwards until the flashes are more or less over. In retrospect the WHI was started so long ago and the doses used were so incredibly high. Nowadays we use much lower doses as a matter of course and if you look at the WHI, the women in the study who used the sorts of HRT regimens we use today did not have the same risk of breast cancer and heart disease.

Their next piece of advice was to try to use HRT for less than five years if possible. That was because it was the five year mark that saw women on combined HRT start to get a big upswing in their rate of breast cancer. Not every woman is through the worst of her night sweats and hot flashes after only five years. In some cases, if the hot flashes continue to wreak havoc with her sleep, the damage done from lack of sleep and the discomfort she feels on a daily basis have to be sorted out. I discuss the pros and cons of continuing the HRT in these women and many choose to roll the dice with the up to 24 per cent increased risk in breast cancer in exchange for decent sleep and the improvement in mood that results.

## Newer studies

In 2012 the results of a much awaited prospective randomized trial called the Kronos Early Estrogen Prevention Study (KEEPS) added fuel to the benefits of HRT in the right circumstances. In this study, women were given low dose combined oestrogen and progesterone in low doses straight after the menopause or a placebo. They found HRT is safe, gives major relief for the symptoms of menopause and improves mood, memory, bone density and the signs of heart disease with no increased risk of breast cancer, stroke or heart attack. They did exclude 'high risk' women for example the very obese, women with known heart disease and heavy smokers. Given that the KEEPS study mimics the way HRT is used today, the results are more reliable for today's woman enduring hot flashes.

## Oestrogen-only HRT

Ok so we know that the feared risks of breast cancer and heart disease are not so alarming if HRT is used at a lower dose, started earlier and if women don't get left on HRT forever. But here's another important mitigating factor; The WHI found that post-menopausal women who took oestrogen-ONLY HRT for six years did NOT increase their risk of death or heart disease. Let be more specific. In the 50s, oestrogen only HRT DECREASED the risk of heart disease. They did find that women who stayed on HRT into their 70s did have a higher risk of heart disease. But very few women need or want to be on HRT in their 70s anyway these days.

As for the risk of breast cancer, in the WHI, the women who took oestrogen only HRT had a slightly LOWER risk of getting breast cancer than women on either combination HRT or no HRT at all.

So with such great statistics, you'd think we'd throw oestrogen-only HRT in the water for all women transitioning into menopause! It's not that simple. The reason we can't use oestrogen-only HRT in most women is that oestrogen causes the endometrium (lining of the uterus) keep building up. You remember from the Hormone Primer that it's the progesterone that packs it down and organizes it. Without the balancing effects of progesterone, the endometrium keeps growing and can either become unhealthily thick or turn to cancer. It's a real risk so we always have to give 'combined' HRT with BOTH oestrogen and progesterone to women with a uterus. However if you've had to have a hysterectomy for another gynaecological problem (see below) you do have the option of oestrogen only HRT.

BOTTOM LINE HRT AND RISK
* HRT is the best treatment for hot flashes, vaginal dryness and menopausal mood swings
* If you start HRT as soon as you get troubled by your hot flashes (either at peri-menopause or once in established menopause), HRT will decrease your risk of heart disease by up to 50 per cent
* HRT significantly reduces the risk of fractures from osteoporosis
* The increased risk of breast cancer on combined HRT is less than 0.1 per cent per year, much less than the increased risks associated with obesity and drinking a single drink of alcohol each day.
* There is a LOWER risk of breast cancer with oestrogen only HRT
* HRT helps prevent dementia

For the final word, I will hand over to the International Menopause Society, who clearly state:

"Healthy women younger than 60 years should not be unduly concerned about the safety profile of HRT. New data and re-analyses of older studies by women's age show that, for most women, the potential benefits of HRT given for a clear indication are many and the risks are few when initiated within a few years of menopause."

Updated IMS recommendations on postmenopausal hormone therapy and preventive strategies for midlife health

CLIMACTERIC 2011;14:302–320

HRT is taken either as tablets or as patches or sometimes a combination of both. It can be 'cyclical', meaning you get a period, just like the pill or continuous, meaning no periods. Cyclical HRT is really only for young women with premature menopause or women in peri-menopause who wish to continue having a 'normal' cycle but are experiencing hot flashes. Most opt for continuous HRT.

### SIDE EFFECTS

Nothing is without side effects. Even though in theory we're just replacing your now dwindling hormone levels, side effects are wide ranging and have been known to put an end to the affair with HRT for some women.

Side effects of oestrogen replacement include;
* Nausea, headaches
* Vaginal bleeding (ugh! Who wants that again?)
* Fluid retention, breast tenderness
* Weight gain (NOT everyone – in fact for most women being menopausal and not taking HRT sees big weight gains!)
* Worsening of some existing conditions such as gallstones, fibroids or in the uterus
* Blood clots

Side effects that come with progesterone replacement;
* Mood swings
* Bloating and diarrhoea
* Headaches

All patches can irritate the skin and some women with sensitive skin just cannot use them.

It's a fact of life that when doctors talk about medications, side effects have to be mentioned because if we gloss over them and you are one of the unlucky few to develop side effects, you can rightly say you didn't have all the information with which to make a good choice for your health. But read the box of a basic paracetamol tablet and the long list of potential side effects are enough to render you a whiter shade of pale. So I mention them in the hope that they won't put you off so much as giving HRT a try if you're suffering from flashes.

With all the mention of side effects and the word cancer being tossed around, no wonder so many women remain really uncomfortable with the whole idea of HRT. Besides, some women feel their symptoms simply aren't bad enough to go down that route. Studies have shown that only 10 to 25 percent of women with menopause symptoms even talk to their doctor about their menopausal problems. And when they do, they're often pretty unhappy with the advice they're given. No wonder then that so many women are looking for an alternative to conventional medicine and HRT to control their symptoms.

So, here is a look at some of the available therapies and what they mean for you and your pesky sleep-stopping flashes:

### BLACK COHOSH

Black cohosh is a herb known as *Actaea racemosa* or *Cimicifuga racemosa*. It is a member of the buttercup family that is native to North America and comes as tablets. We don't know how it works. Studies on hormone levels show they don't move on this herb so that to the extent that they work to combat hot flashes, they're not working through boosting oestrogen levels. Studies on Black Cohosh's ability to curb hot flashes are a mixed bag. Many smaller studies did find some positive results but other studies have tended to find no advantage over placebo. All the studies are hamstrung by a lack of scientific rigour making strict interpretation difficult. In my experience, it doesn't touch the sides of hot flashes when they're anything other than mild. And women with mild hot flashes tend to grin and bear them rather than taking anything for them. But they remain very popular despite the fact that they aren't much chop.

Generally black cohosh is pretty safe. Some women get headaches and tummy pains, but they're not common. There are worrying reports of liver damage at therapeutic doses but of the millions of women who take it around the world, it's still a rare event. Regardless, The Australian Therapeutic Goods Administration has ordered that Black cohosh packages come with a warning about the risk of liver damage printed on the box. It's the only country in the world with that warning.

### Soy proteins

We know that Asian diets are high in soy-based foods and that women living in these countries express few menopausal complaints as well as less heart disease and breast cancer. It is unknown if the lower prevalence of hot flashes and other menopausal symptoms are due to dietary make-up, cultural factors, or a combination of both, but soy proteins have become very popular as the elixirs of health.

Recently a complementary therapist gave me a stern talking to about the dangers of high tofu diet. So I thought I should address some concerns you might have or some of the scarier aspects of soy foods you might have heard;

Soy foods, such as tofu and soy milk contain phytoestrogens. These chemicals activate some oestrogen receptors in the body. That's raised alarm bells with some scientists. After all anything that mucks around with oestrogen receptors is potentially dangerous, right? Infertility, early puberty and other hormone issues have been hypothesized. It sounds terrible! In reality, there's no evidence a diet high in tofu and tempeh (or even in soy proteins that make up the bulk of protein drinks and bars!) is harmful. BUT – and there is a but... Feeding soy milk and formula to babies is another story with some studies pointing to a possible link to infertility and early puberty. For now, for women in the menopause can consider upping soy consumption and seeing how that goes for you.

### Lose weight

An enormous US study of menopausal women yielded an unexpected result.

Weight loss emerged as an excellent treatment for hot flashes! For the women suffering from flashes, losing ten or more percent of their body weight was enough to eliminate the flashes altogether in many of the women, and significantly reduce the symptoms in the others. Bottom line; if looking hot, not needing to fork out for a new 'fat' wardrobe and disease reduction weren't enough reason to try diet and exercise, maybe the tantalising prospect of nuking your flashes will be!

### ACUPUNCTURE

There have been many studies on acupuncture for hot flashes. Most of them have been poorly funded and small and it's been difficult to know how broadly to interpret the results. In that vein, in 2009 there was a review of the 19 studies that had been done to that point and the results of all of them were analysed. The bottom line: no evidence that it works. But before you fall in a heap and go back to the drawing board, the reviewers did point out that the results were promising, the only problem was the lack of scientific rigour of the studies. It may work for you and there are few side effects from acupuncture. So why not give it a shot? Your worst case scenario is that it's a waste of time and money.

### EXERCISE

There's a benefit seen with exercise. Good news or bad news? I guess that depends on your perspective but the fact is it is a great way to manage your sleep post menopause. A large Finnish study of post menopausal women who were still having hot flashes found that after six months of aerobics classes, women's hot flashes and night sweats had reduced by 20 per cent.

### YOGA

Take everything I just said about acupuncture and repeat it, this time for yoga. In 2009 Korean researchers reviewed 14 studies for yoga and hot flashes finding the results 'unconvincing'. Once again, though, it was the poor quality of the studies, rather than negative results per se that led to a lack of evidence to support yoga. As with acupuncture there is no harm from yoga, in fact it is a brilliant stress buster and awesome for posture and back pain. Plus, it is a work out, and as we're all about pushing exercise in this book, I think worst-case scenario you will get a work out and still need some help from HRT!

### MASSAGE

Now you're listening! Who doesn't benefit from a massage? An Iranian study of massage, especially if accompanied by some essential oils (the oils studied were lavender, rose, rosemary, almond and evening primrose) found improvements in almost every symptom of menopause. The authors of the study themselves were wary of concluding too much because there were only 90 women in the study and it's not the kind of thing you can control for with a placebo. But massage is relaxing and it just goes to show how stress can make symptoms, including hot flashes, worse. So anything that relaxes you can help beyond simply addressing the mess in your mind.

### HYPNOSIS

In a study of 187 postmenopausal women who reported having at least seven hot flashes a day, half the women were given five 45-minute training sessions in self-hypnosis and the other half had five counselling sessions without hypnosis. The women kept a diary of their flashes.

And just 12 weeks later, women in the hypnosis group reported 74 per cent fewer hot flashes on average, compared with 17 per cent fewer among the women who just had counselling. Plus hypnosis significantly reduced the chances of waking at night from flashes.

A single small study does not a positive conclusion make. But hypnosis is unlikely to be harmful so feel free to give it a go.

### TIBOLONE

Tibolone is a fascinating drug. It is referred to as an 'oestrogen alternative' and works like hormone replacement therapy with a difference. On its own its effects on the body are minimal. But once it passes through the guts and gets broken down in the liver, the break-down products travel through the blood stream to various target organs and the effects on the oestrogen receptors in each are slightly different. For a start, it is excellent at decreasing hot flashes. It's not as effective as HRT but comes a close second. It also acts on the vagina, making it moister, plus because it is also partially broken down into testosterone, it can help with libido and enjoying your time in the bedroom (See Are My Hormones

Destroying My Libido?). It also helps build bones and prevent osteoporosis. But it doesn't give you the usual oestrogen effects on the uterus and doesn't cause breast tenderness.

Tibolone shows no increased risk of clotting, unlike oestrogen. Initially, it looked like it might actually lower the risk of breast cancer because one large trial, called the LIFT trial, suggested as much. That got everyone really excited! But a subsequent trial of tibolone in menopausal women who had suffered breast cancer found that it increased the risk of recurrence of breast cancers. That threw the kibosh on that theory and now everybody shrugs their shoulders and says we don't know the effect on breast cancer, but it shouldn't be used on women who have had breast cancer in the past.

If you have an intact uterus, you should not take tibolone until it has been a year since your last period. Taking it earlier than that can cause some irregular breakthrough bleeding. If you're already on HRT, you can simply switch over to tibolone at any time. . If you've had a hysterectomy, there's no need to wait. You can start straight away. If you're on tibolone and get some break through bleeding, see your doctor.

### FISH OIL

Bit of a lack of hard core evidence, once again, I'm afraid. One study found that women with menopausal hot flashes benefited from taking EPA (one of the healthy omega-3 fatty acids found in fish oil) as a supplement. The supplement reduced the number (but not the severity) of hot flashes. The side benefit is, of course, the potential prevention of heart disease and as you transition through menopause that becomes more important than ever.

### ANTI-DEPRESSANTS

After HRT, taking these medicines are the next most effective step you can take to control hot flashes. Patients who are put into menopause medically (or surgically) especially because they have breast cancer often rely on them. The most effective one is venlafaxine. They work by increasing the levels of a chemical called serotonin in your brain. This seems to help regulate your body temperature, although exactly how isn't completely understood yet. For free, taking venlafaxine should help with the mood swings that can also accompany menopause (See Are My Hormones Making Me Moody?)

They're not without side effects. They can cause dizziness, nausea and light-headedness. They can also wreak havoc with your libido and your ability to achieve a climax in the bedroom. To top it off, some women get a rise in the blood pressure from them as well.

Plus while studies have shown you can expect a brilliant 60 per cent reduction in the number and severity of your flashes, you are unlikely to nix them altogether. Plus for my patients, if they're not prepared to take HRT, they often have similar reservations about antidepressants.

## BIO-IDENTICAL HORMONES FOR MENOPAUSE

The great debate continues. After the Women's Health Initiative study results came out we saw an explosion of 'Bio-Identical Hormone Therapy' businesses all over the world. They're basically hormones that are compounded by a lab to be identical in molecular structure to the hormones women make naturally in their bodies. The oestrogens are made using plant chemicals extracted from yams and soy. Bio-identical progesterone is micronized (finely ground) in the laboratory for better absorption in the body. Doctors who prescribe bio-identical hormones say that they can tailor your hormones to suit your individual needs, rather than pulling them out of a pre-packaged bag.

There are claims that bio-identical hormones, while they are a form of hormone replacement therapy, are safer than conventional HRT. Lots of women saw Oprah chiming in on TV and extolling the virtues of her bio-identical hormone experience and lots of my girlfriends and patients have tried it. However, to many doctors, these things are potentially dangerous. Let me explain their concerns:

**The claim:** Bio-identical hormones are made from a natural oestrogen. On lots of websites you will read that conventional HRT is made out of horse urine. Bio-identical oestrogens are a combination of oestradiol, oestriol and oestrone (see the Hormone Primer to refresh your memory on the types of oestrogen). It is a big part of the bio-identical sales pitch, claiming this mixture is this spe-

82

cial, unique blend of oestrogens that replicates more naturally what is in your body.

**The truth:** Old fashioned conventional oestrogens were made out of oestrogens obtained from the urine of pregnant mares. Those conjugated oestrogens are less popular these days. We use 'micronised' (finely ground) synthetic oestradiol these days. Bio-identical hormones tend to use micronised progestogens made from diosgenin from yams. Not sure how bio-identical I am to a yam. But I think there's a hair's breadth between bio-identical and the synthetic version. There's no evidence the body can distinguish between them. By the way, if you don't chemically alter a yam to get progestogen, and just shove yam cream on your leg, (and there are lots of yam creams advertised on the net for flashes!!) you get zero effect.

In terms of the different types of oestrogens, the Australian Menopause Centre says that it doesn't matter what form of oestrogens you take as they're all converted to the same form once they get into your body. If you remember, Oestradiol is the one that is made by the ovaries and is the most potent type of oestrogen. It is the one that you will be missing most when menopause hits. So as for using a combination with oestriol and oestrone, I'm not sure you need the weak menopausal or pregnancy oestrogen anyway?

**The claim:** Often you will have some tests to tailor-make a hormone cocktail to your body's needs. The tests use salivary and some blood tests.

**The truth:** The scientific evidence to support these types of tests is definitely growing but often the labs themselves aren't regulated properly. That's the reason their results are often rejected by more conventional doctors.

**The claim:** Bio-identical hormones are safer than conventional HRT.

**The truth:** You wouldn't know because a) They're not studied for long-term effects and b) They're not regulated by any government body.

You have no idea what is in an unregulated product. For example, according to one British report, 2 oz jars of Progest cream (a commercial preparation of bio-identical progesterone cream advertised for menopausal symptoms) used in a clinical trial contained 100 mg progesterone per ounce rather than the 465 mg claimed by the manufacturer. It's a matter of buyer beware. There could be dangerous contaminants, animal parts, there could be bacterial overgrowth or any number of safety issues with these products.

Even the products prescribed by doctors who are well trained can be problematic. I trust most pharmacists to be ethical and to compound a prescription exactly as the doctor has written it. But without government oversight, it is not guaranteed. With hormone treatments bought on the internet, all bets are off and you should assume that the chasm between what's advertised and what's delivered is huge!

I have another concern. You often see the oestrogen mixtures combined with a cocktail of other bio-identical hormones like testosterone, DHEA, growth hormone, pregnenolone, thyroxine and melatonin. You can't just go taking hormones you don't need without medical supervision. That can spell trouble. For example, you can throw your thyroid into a spin if your own levels are fine and you start propping it up with supplemental hormones. DHEA, testosterone and pregnenolone are not approved by the FDA for women

Having said all of that
  * Lots of women find these treatments effective in a way that traditional HRT never was for them.
  * In the hands of a good doctor and pharmacist, they can be excellent
  * Lack of studies doesn't mean that these products ARE harmful, just that we can't guarantee safety.

So, bottom line, my advice is this:
  * NEVER, ever, ever buy anything off the internet and treat yourself
  * Only a doctor should put you on compounded tailored hormone treatments if you are going to use them.
  * Go into bio-identical hormones armed with the knowledge that their safety and efficacy cannot be guaranteed.

# Are my hormones giving me sleep apnoea?

Another possible missing link between menopause and insomnia and fatigue is sleep apnoea, which does affect 6.5 per cent of women aged 30–39 years. But this figure rises to 16 per cent of women aged 50–60 years). In sleep apnoea, your upper airways around your throat collapse during your sleep so that you snore in an increasing volume as the minutes tick on and have moments (for anywhere between 15 and 90 seconds at a time) where you stop breathing altogether. Your body responds by forcefully opening up your airways with a fairly dramatic and loud snore and then the whole snoring crescendo starts over again. If you tend to wake up feeling like you've hardly slept at all and / or your partner complains about your snoring, you should think about whether you could have sleep apnoea. Other clues include having problems concentrating and remembering things during the day, or you might wake up with a headache and can be a moody witch as well. Sleep apnoea is more likely if you are overweight and if you tend to like an evening drink.

Blame your hormones? Yep! Menopause triggers the start of sleep apnoea in many women. That might be because of the post-menopausal weight gain but doctors also think that the lower progesterone levels play a role as well because progesterone stimulates breathing.

If you are reading this and nodding, or if you think it simply MIGHT be a possibility in your case, you should book an appointment with your GP and raise the prospect of sleep apnoea. Diagnosing it involves being monitored during your sleep. You used to have to go to a lab and get hooked up to a truckload of monitors. It was either extremely expensive or involved the waiting list from hell to get the test done on the public list. Lately I have been referring patients for a home sleep apnoea test. They send you all the equipment and instructions and you simply send everything back and they give you a diagnosis. It's so easy! Ask your GP if you think that sounds like a good option for you.

# How to handle your sleep apnoea

It is important to treat sleep apnoea because besides making you feel like ten tons of rubbish, there's a hefty link to heart disease.

### LIFESTYLE CHANGES
Given that being overweight and drinking too much alcohol are both linked to developing sleep apnoea, there is general advice all patients will get: Losing some weight and cutting down alcohol is the first port of call. Studies have linked both interventions to big improvements in sleep apnoea symptoms. All doctors should recommend this as step one through twenty with other options only considered after that.

### SPECIAL EQUIPMENT
The second step (assuming you can't or it doesn't get rid of the problem altogether) is getting fitted with a CPAP mask. CPAP stands for Continuous Positive Airways pressure. It is a little machine which uses positive pressure to hold your airways open. The CPAP is applied either through a mask that fits over your nose and mouth or just the nose. It sounds ghastly but it is amazingly well tolerated by most people.

### LAST RESORT
The last step is surgery. Uvulopalatopharyngoplasty is surgery to open up the upper airways by removing excess tissue such as the uvula (the dangly bit that hangs down at the back of the throat), part of the soft palate and possibly other tissues in that vicinity. As a stand-alone procedure without CPAP or weight loss and alcohol reduction it has pretty poor data to recommend it. Success rates are around 40 per cent, but unfortunately, by the two-year mark many if not most patients are back to square one. Discuss this with your GP before you make any moves towards surgery. I tend to try talk my patients out of it.

# Is heavy bleeding making me tired?

We have hit one of the most common hormonal problems I see in women in their mid to late 40s as well as young teens, heavy bleeding. It's not something we women talk about, even to our doctor. We tend to simply expect to bleed heavily at the age when menopause is approaching and so we don't discuss it. But heavy periods can wreak havoc with your body.

I can't tell you how many of my women patients at either end of the menstrual era (either youngish teens or late 40s) come in with some general complaint which smacks of an iron issue and sure enough when I run blood tests, they reveal shocking iron deficiency. It's then that I ask the question about periods and hear the sorry tales of heavy bleeding, overflowing, clots and exhaustion.

Heavy menstrual bleeding can take a heavy toll on women. For a start, losing blood means losing iron. Iron is at the heart of the haemoglobin molecule that carries oxygen around to the tissues. Not enough iron? Expect to have your cells starved of oxygen. But it's not just that these women are running around with stupidly low iron levels and not functioning properly, it's that this bleeding takes an emotional toll as well. It is often unpredictable. It is so heavy it can be embarrassing. It can make it hard to function at work and at home.

But first let's deal with the iron deficiency itself. What are my super sleuth clues to iron deficiency? They're not actually that hard to pick... If you are low in iron you will probably feel exhausted and weak, you will have a dodgy immune system and catch more little infections. You may feel the cold and feel light-headed. In more severe cases you might experience a rapid heartbeat and shortness of breath when you exercise.

## About Iron

So while I am talking about iron deficiency, I should explain that not all iron deficiency is necessarily hormonal and caused by bleeding. Iron levels in your body are a product of two things; iron in and iron out. Let's start with iron in. There are two kinds of dietary iron, haem and non-haem. Haem iron is efficiently absorbed from your guts but is only found in meat, fish and chicken (or other poultry). Non-haem iron is the stuff you find in vegetables, 'fortified' foods (like the breads and breakfast cereals with iron added in), iron supplements that you buy over the counter from the pharmacy and acidic foods cooked in cast-iron pots.

The distinction is important because while 15 to 30 per cent of haem iron that you eat is absorbed, that number is only 5 per cent for non-haem iron. That is why many if not most vegetarians will need a supplement.

Then there are other factors that can affect how much iron you absorb through your guts. Some vegetables and herbs like spinach, chives and parsley contain oxalic acid which interferes with iron absorption. Another group of culprits that stops iron absorption are some high-fibre foods like pulses (lentils and the like) and wholegrains that contain chemicals known as phytates, which plants use to store phosphorous. In the enormous Framingham study, people who ate more than seven servings of wholegrains each week had the lowest levels of iron. That's a crying shame because in so many ways, the high grain diet is so good. Phytates not only bind iron, but will bind zinc, calcium and magnesium as well and stop them from being absorbed properly. And bringing up the rear, foods high in calcium like dairy also reduce the amount of iron that enters blood.

On the flip side, vitamin C and other acids naturally present in fruits (especially oranges, papayas and peaches) fruit juices (especially orange juice) and some vegetables like red capsicum, broccoli and Brussels sprouts) increase iron absorption.

So here's the low down from me; I have never met anyone whose iron deficiency resulted from too much wholegrain food and dairy and not enough orange juice. But eating in an iron-healthy way does start to matter when we're trying to get your iron levels up.

I'm going to come out here as a non-meat eater. It's not religious. It's just that I don't particularly like red meat. Also, I think the carbon footprint of animals reared for eating is too high and on a purely personal level, I happen to really like animals. We have two gorgeous dogs and I just can't bring myself to eat a living creature that has died simply for my meal. I don't judge anyone who doesn't feel that, but to me, I simply don't want to EAT an animal. Don't ask for logic because I find it easy to EAT fish. I just don't find my heart moved by the death of a fish.

Recently I had a blood test and I guess, not surprisingly, my GP ordered an iron test. I was worried. I have never had an iron supplement but technically my diet is pretty iron unfriendly. Turns out I shouldn't have been too stressed. My ferritin was 49 (more on the significance of these numbers soon). It was much, MUCH higher than many if not most of my patients. Which goes to show that a healthy meat-free diet can give you plenty of iron without you having to take a pill.

But for most people, red meat is the key to iron from a consumption perspective. In another study by the Framingham researchers, men and women aged 68 to 93 had the highest levels of stored iron if they consumed red meat four or more times a week, took more than 30 milligrams of an iron supplement daily, or ate more than 21 servings of fruit each week. However, levels were much lower among those who consumed more than seven servings of wholegrains each week. Now before you head to the local butcher and get over-enthusiastic with red meat as your new staple, there are some real risks with having too much of it. Remember: "moderation" (in the case of red meat that means no more than three serves per week). More than three serves per week of red meat has been linked to both bowel cancer and strokes.

But for most of my patients who are iron deficient, not eating enough iron is a part of the problem but not the whole story. The issue is they're losing iron through the blood. It's leaving the station somewhere and the doctor's job is to find out where from. In men, the elderly or even children, unexplained blood loss needs to be investigated. That's because you can get a slow leak from your guts or from the urinary system (bladder or kidneys) that is small enough to go undetected. By now most of us know to look for blood in the toilet bowl. But blood oxidises so that after exposure to oxygen, red blood turns dark brown, or if there's enough of it, it looks black. In fact red blood in your toilet bowl probably tells you that the blood is coming from your anus. The two major culprits are haemorrhoids (basically varicose veins in your back passage that tend to bleed after a bowel motion) or an anal fissure, which is a tear in the bottom, usually because of constipation and the need to pass a very hard brick like poo!

But blood can leak from a stomach ulcer or an exposed vein in what we call an erosion with no symptoms. The oxidised blood just makes the poo a darker colour but is so mixed in you would never see it as blood.

For the purposes of this book on hormones, I'm going to assume that this is not the case. Because we don't need to go into all the things that go into diagnosing and treating this problem here and now. What I do want to discuss is heavy periods, as in my experience, it is the cause of so many problems for women and unless you raise it with your GP, you might live with this issue far longer and with far more devastating consequences than necessary.

### So what's normal?

Random fact of the day: a normal menstrual cycle is 21–35 days per cycle, and normal bleeding lasts an average of seven days and flow measures between 25 and 80 ml. Over 80 in flow earns you the dubious diagnosis of MENORRHAGIA (or heavy periods). No, I don't expect you to measure it. We can usually tell by chatting to you. I always ask about blood clots. Clots are not normal in a period and tell me your flow is too heavy.

# Hormonal causes of heavy bleeding

### Anovulation (not ovulating)

If you head back to our hormone primer, you will see how incredibly complex the menstrual cycle is. From a hormone perspective there are so many opportunities for things to go wrong, it's amazing so many women go most of their fertile lives with a 28-day regular cycle! At the start of your fertile life and at the end, your hypothalamus and pituitary are working pretty normally but your ovaries don't perform as well.

Once you enter the peri-menopause everything starts to change. Your FSH doesn't get your slightly worn out follicles to develop as well as they used to, resulting in a lacklustre production of oestrogen. There's enough oestrogen around to get a nice thick lining on the uterus (endometrium.) But the suboptimal follicles do not respond to an LH surge and as a result they do not ovulate and you don't get a corpus luteum. No corpus luteum means no progesterone. No progesterone means no maturation of the endometrium. This is what we call 'unopposed oestrogen'. You get a thick overblown endometrium but it's disorganized. When it finally outgrows its blood supply and degenerates, you get this chaotic breakdown of the endometrial lining at different levels. That is why 'anovulatory' bleeding is heavier than normal periods. For some women, it can feel like life is just one long period. Periods can start lasting two weeks at a time!

It's not dissimilar when you're first getting into a regular cycle when you first hit puberty. Until the ovaries and brain click into the hormonal rhythm, it can take a while for a regular cycle to establish. Immature follicles can also fail to produce enough oestrogen to achieve a nice follicle and just like happens at the end of your reproductive life, ovulation doesn't occur.

So if you remember being 13 and starting to get your periods and flooding, or you are in your late 40s and suddenly your periods have become monstrous, clotty gushes, chances are you were (and now are) not ovulating. In the case of young girls, the menstrual system works out what it's doing pretty quickly and normal ovulatory cycles start within a few months. For those of us at the end of our hormonal lives, I can't tell you how long it will take. It can last for years, by which time your iron stores are on their knees and you are feeling exhausted all the time. You can't continue to gush blood and not run out of iron at some point.

You need to see your GP first of all to rule out another cause of the heavy bleeding (see below) and to get your iron levels measured.

## How to handle your hormonal heavy bleeding

Your GP may try a non-steroidal anti-inflammatory drug such as diclofenac or ibuprofen. Studies show that you can slow down heavy menstrual blood flow by up to 50 per cent.

A really popular treatment is progestin. Progestins basically balance out the oestrogen in the endometrium stopping the endometrium from over growing and making it more organised and packed down. You can take tablets two to three times a day from days five to 26 of your menstrual cycle, counting the first day of your period as day one. They're not contraceptive though. You can also get progestin as an injection. But weight gain is a side effect that puts many women off.

Or you can get fitted with an IUD that slowly releases artificial progesterone called levonorgestrel (the Mirena). You will remember meeting this one in the Hormone Primer. This type of IUD slows down menstrual blood loss by as much as 97 per cent. I love the Mirena because it is such an effective contraception, plus it slows your periods down unbelievably and some women just need a panty liner for three days instead of Super Maxi tampons every hour for 10 days. Great for your iron stores. Plus I love the set and forget part of it. Get it inserted and you don't have to think about contraception for five years. Initially you can get a bit of spotting for a couple of months until it settles in but I always advise my patients to persist because it's worth it.

Lastly, going on the pill to thin the endometrium is a popular way to go. Often you need reasonably high doses of hormones at the end of your fertile life. The advantages of the pill include the contraceptive effect as well as regulating the cycle which is a huge issue for young girls. Plus in young girls it often makes period pains more bearable.

Surgery is your last resort. Gynaecologists will sometimes suggest a dilatation and curettage (D&C). The gynaecologist scrapes out the lining of the uterus. It's really best for getting a diagnosis. The gynaecologist sends off a sample of the endometrium to the lab to make sure there's no cancer or adenomyosis (see below). It is a pretty hopeless treatment because it typically tends to work for only one or two months at most.

If they don't think a pathology sample is needed, they'll usually opt for something called an endometrial ablation where they basically zap the endometrium. This can be done using laser, heat, ice or an electric current all while you are under a general anaesthetic. Once the endometrium is 'ablated', you are starting from scratch and hopefully the hormonal issues can be sorted out with a new beginning in the uterus! Hysterectomy is only used if there is something else going on. As you will see, when things go haywire in the peri-menopause, there is OFTEN something else going on! I'll go through the most common 'something elses' I see....

### Fibroids (leiomyomas)

Around one in five women has at least one fibroid during their fertile years but once you hit peri-menopause, that number booms out so that by 50, half of us have them! Fibroids are benign tumours in the muscle of the uterus and although you can get one at a time, they tend to be clustered. We don't know what causes them, except that they are hormonal and tend to be fuelled by oestrogen so when you pass through menopause they either stop growing or shrink. They can be so tiny you need a microscope to see them (in which case you will never be worried by them) or they can be enormous – even up to a kilo in weight.

Only one in four women gets symptoms. They tend to be around the bulky size if they're large, so a dragging pain in the pelvic area, painful sex and maybe needing to pee all the time as the extra weight presses on the bladder. But more common are symptoms around bleeding: heavy, prolonged and irregular bleeding. The reason they cause heavy bleeding is that they can disrupt a blood vessel by growing into it.

We know some things increase your chances of getting fibroids, like eating more red meat and that eating more fish, green veggies and fruit helps protect you from getting them. But once you have them and they're making you bleed, the bleeding is unlikely to stop until you get them sorted or reach full blown menopause. Most women opt for treatment because besides spending their life drained of iron, the constant bleeding is a pain in the neck.

Fibroids are diagnosed on an ultrasound scan.

The first line in treatment is often the same Mirena as we use for anovulatory bleeding. The tiny amount of progestin released by the Mirena stabilises the lining of the uterus and sorts out the bleeding. The alternatives are basically all surgical. You'll need a referral to a gynaecologist. Your options include getting the artery that feeds it injected with a substance that cuts off the fibroid's blood supply, which makes it shrink (arterial embolisation), or having them removed. The arterial embolisation is brilliant if you're young and still want a family so you can't part with your uterus but fibroids are contributing to heavy bleeding, pain or infertility. You need a highly qualified specialist in the field and it's not cheap.

Surgically removing individual fibroids can be a really simple operation, but it does depend a bit on where they're located. Plus if you have lots of big ones, it is a bit more difficult surgery. So if you no longer need a uterus for child bearing purposes and removing the fibroids is an issue, you might be offered a hysterectomy, (see below).

### Uterine Polyps

These are basically benign overgrowths of the endometrial cells that form a little growth that project into the cavity of the uterus. They can be tiny, around a millimetre in diameter, to about the size of a golf ball or occasionally even bigger and they hang off a thin stalk from the endometrium. Exactly like fibroids, we don't know why they happen, but do know that they have something to do with oestrogen, which makes them grow. Polyps cause heavy bleeding as they grow because they dangle from their stalks and rub on and irritate the endometrium they touch, which ultimately rubs off the endometrium and exposes the little blood vessels underneath.

As with fibroids, they tend to shrink after the menopause and, like fibroids, they tend to crop up around the end of your fertile life in the 40s. They're more common in overweight ladies, especially those with high blood pressure. I will sometimes see them when doing a pap smear. My patients nearly keel over when I mention it to them.

Like fibroids, unless they're visible on the cervix (like the women whose polyps I see when I'm doing a pap test) they tend to be found on an ultrasound scan when we're looking for the cause of irregular or heavy bleeding or bleeding after sex.

Rarely, they can turn cancerous. RARELY. But it does happen and for this reason, most gynaecologists suggest having them removed, especially if they're causing you bleeding anyway. It usually requires a general anaesthetic and surgery BUT it can be done through the opening of the cervix without any scars.

### Adenomyosis

This is a whacky disease where the endometrium starts growing into the wall of the uterus. It's a variation on endometriosis where the endometrium starts growing out of the uterus altogether, on the ovaries, tubes, bowel... all over the place! If the adenomyosis just happens in one single spot, it is called an adenomyoma.

Like fibroids and polyps, it's a problem of the late 40s just before the menopause. It causes heavy bleeding and tends to disappear after menopause when your oestrogen reserves are depleted. And once again we don't know what causes it.

Where it differs from the other conditions, though is that it will tend to be painful because the endometrium sloughs off during the period but the blood is trapped inside the uterine wall and causes pain. Women with adenomyosis get heavy, painful periods starting in their late 30s or early 40s. In fact, if you could take all the uteruses that have been removed by hysterectomy where pain was a symptom and check them out under a microscope, adenomyosis is there in up to a quarter of them.

You can only diagnose it 100 per cent by looking at the uterus tissue under a microscope. Which means removing the uterus by hysterectomy. The history of heavy, painful periods is suggestive, as is the finding of a large, slightly tender uterus on examination, and sometimes there are suggestive features on an ultrasound. But the final ultimate diagnosis only comes after a pathologist has a good look at the uterus itself.

Your doctor might try using non steroidal anti-inflammatory drugs like diclofenac or ibuprofen or some progestogens like we use for anovulatory bleeding, but if these don't work, you might be looking at a hysterectomy. If you're freaking out about that, keep reading....

## A note about hysterectomy

Seen as a barbaric butchery of women, removing the uterus is almost taboo nowadays. If I drop the 'H bomb' on my patients (suggest they may need a hysterectomy), a goodly number will run screaming from the room (well not literally but you know what I mean.) Many of us have heard the dark family folklore that says that grandma was never the same after her hysterectomy. Some doctor (no doubt male) hacked off the heart of her femininity and she never recovered.

So here I will declare why at the first sign of something unseemly happening with my secret women's business, I will be heading to my gynaecologist and begging for a hysterectomy. Sure it's surgery. Sure it needs a general anaesthetic. Sure it is not free of risk... so here's why I'm planning my hysterectomy if I need it:

* It will COMPLETELY relieve for good whatever nasty bleeding or pain I am having. (Not that I'm having it yet but I'm thinking ahead!) Whether I cop fibroids, adenomyosis or

just heavy anovulatory bleeding, it will be fixed for good.
* I can have HRT for longer. Without a uterus I can avail myself of oestrogen-only HRT, safe in the knowledge that not only will I avoid hot flashes, sexual issues, dry vagina and mood swings, but I will not increase my risk of heart disease or breast cancer. Plus less wrinkles, less unsightly body hair, less hair loss on my head!! Yeah!!! Bring it on!!!!!
* There will be no more need for pap tests. No cervix means no pap tests. A minor thing but hey, why not!!??
* There is a lower ovarian cancer risk – for ALL hysterectomy patients
* There will be no more need to worry about cervical or uterine cancer. If you ain't got a cervix or uterus, you can't get cancer on 'em.

## Myths about hysterectomy

* You're out of action for six weeks. My patients generally stay in hospital for one to three nights (average is two). They're back to driving a week later, back to work in around three weeks and feeling like nothing ever happened after four weeks.
* You become menopausal and grouchy. Generally the ovaries are left inside. You will get whatever oestrogen they're producing. But for most women, their menopause is nigh anyway, which is why they're having issues with that part of the anatomy in the first place.
* Prolapse of the uterus. This is another piece of secret women's business that we don't discuss. The pelvic floor is just a sling of muscles that supports your bladder, uterus and lower bowel. They rest on this muscle band, which holds them up and out of the vagina. If the pelvic floor is slack, the organs I've listed can slip down and bulge into the vagina. You might feel a bit of a lump or something uncomfortable in your vagina and often you can get lots of urine infections and leakage of urine. Your pelvic floor often gets completely smashed by labour and then menopause adds another issue into the mix. That's because oestrogen keeps the pelvic floor well

supplied by blood and therefore makes it nice and strong. The link between hysterectomy and prolapsed uterus is not so much a myth as a bit of an outdated fact.

* In the old days of straightforward abdominal hysterectomy or even vaginal hysterectomy (when the gynaecologist removed the uterus via the vagina instead of out the tummy wall), the gynaecologist had to slice through a critical part of the pelvic floor, the 'utero-sacral ligaments' to get the uterus out. A higher risk of prolapse was a problem with hysterectomy although it didn't happen until around 20 years after the operation. These days with laparoscopic hysterectomy (keyhole surgery) cutting the utero-sacral ligament isn't required. There are enormous studies on at the moment to evaluate the risk of prolapse but because it is a relatively new procedure, we don't have hard data. But reports from the surgeons at the hospital I refer into suggest that prolapsed uterus is unlikely to be an issue with the new procedure.

# Fixing your tiredness caused by heavy bleeding

Of course, apart from finding the cause of your excess bleeding, we have to look at the effects and, primarily, that's going to be fixing your iron levels.

We have to replace the iron you're losing and there are a few ways we can do that:

## IRON TABLETS

Iron tablets are cheap, easy and don't hurt. But they can make you constipated and bloated and because they're non-haem iron, they get absorbed slowly, which means it can take a while to bring your levels up. They're fine for mild iron deficiency. But for lots of my patients with peri-menopausal bleeding, they are really, really low in iron and the tablets will take too long to get them feeling right again.

## IRON INJECTIONS

Owwwww! Looking at a vial of iron, they're HUGE and most women who have had these injections have found them to be painful.

It was actually our practice nurse, Sister Muriel Baird, a veteran of women's health who showed me how easy and painless it can be to use iron injections. She mixes the vial with half a millilitre of local anaesthetic and injects the lot. Few of my patients report pain with this technique. I do weekly iron injections of two vials at a time and this is often enough to fix the problem.

IRON INFUSION

In this method, ten vials of iron are run into the vein through a drip. Most GPs don't have the infrastructure to do this so I refer to my local private haematologist who will take patients with a very low iron level and perform the infusion in his rooms. You need to take a day off work and many people get a fever or an allergic reaction from such a massive dose at once. But once it's all in, you don't have to come back each week for more shots.

You need a good two weeks for injected iron to be fully integrated into your haemoglobin and carrying a full load of oxygen again. So if you think after a single iron injection you will walk out of the surgery feeling like you're zinging, think again. It's a nice, slow recovery of your energy levels and ability to concentrate that's in order here!

Fixing peri-menopausal bleeding and giving iron deficient women iron is one of the most satisfying things I do in my practice. Explaining to these exhausted women that there's a reason they're feeling so old and exhausted and seeing them turn around and feel ten years younger so quickly is one of the best things I can do as a doctor.

But you should always have medical supervision when taking iron supplements because you can get too much of a good thing....

A NOTE ABOUT TOO MUCH IRON

There is one tiny problem with iron. Aside from bleeding, the body doesn't have an easy way to get rid of it, if it starts building up. Too much iron isn't great for the body as the excess iron gets shoved into your liver, heart and pancreas, where it can ultimately lead to cirrhosis, liver cancer, heart rhythm problems and diabetes.

There is a genetic disease called haemochromatosis, where people tend to accumulate very high levels of stored iron. But even for people without haemochromatosis, high iron can still be a problem. One huge study of 32,000 women who were followed healthwise for 10 years was the Nurses' Health Study. It is often quoted because we have accumulated so much data from these 32,000 women. Well, it found that the women with the highest iron levels were nearly three times as likely to get diabetes as those with the lowest iron levels. There was another huge study called the Health Professionals Follow-up Study, which followed 38,000 men and once again, the guys who ate the most haem iron had a 63 per cent higher risk of diabetes than the men with the lowest iron intake.

And there are a few studies that have shown that people with high levels of iron who regularly donate blood increase their insulin sensitivity and lower their risk of diabetes.

As I tell my mum all the time (as she tries to force-feed me a steak telling me avoiding red meat isn't natural), heavy red meat consumption is linked to bowel (and prostate) cancer and some people believe it is the excess iron consumption that is the problem. While most people agree the link between heavy red meat consumption and heart disease and stroke is more likely to be exposure to more saturated fats than more iron.

So, before you think taking a hit of iron sounds like a bright idea, only do so under medical supervision. Get your iron levels tested before taking a supplement because it is possible to do more harm than good.

# Are polycystic ovaries and insulin resistance making me tired?

Polycystic Ovarian Syndrome and insulin resistance are conditions that go hand in hand and stuff up everything. I have allotted quite a lot of space to these problems in Are My Hormones Making Me Fat? That's because rapid and immovable weight gain is often one of the primary symptoms.

Briefly, in this condition, there is an inability to properly handle carbohydrates because your insulin receptors do not work effectively. This sets up a cascade of hormonal problems which leave you with a random combination of weight gain, acne, hairiness on your body but hair loss from your head, mood swings, heavy and irregular periods, infertility, a tendency to miscarry and fatigue.

The link between this condition and fatigue is the ineffective transfer of sugar from the blood stream into the cells, where they are needed for fuel. As a result, people with this condition often find it difficult to concentrate – and they feel tired and light-headed, especially in the afternoons.

Sugar cravings can be dreadful as your starving cells put out the call for more sugar.

Many will suffer from serious low sugar attacks and feel light-headed, trembly, sweaty and irritable. These are the people with a subset of insulin resistance known as Type B syndrome. It is an immune system issue. They have a sudden sugar drop because of an interaction between an abnormal antibody in their blood stream and their insulin receptors. These antibodies effectively block the receptors and stop insulin from attaching itself. The abnormal antibodies tend to all fall off in a sudden bang allowing the MASSES of accumulated insulin in your blood onto the receptors, so you get a FLOOD of sugar into the cells. That causes a drop in the blood sugar, also known as hypoglycemia.

Keep reading the rest of this book because I will tell you more about PCOS and IR at every chapter and it might indicate that you need to be diagnosed with and treated for this condition.

# If not hormones then what?

Not all causes of tiredness are hormonal and no look at tiredness would be complete without at least looking at some of the other things you should consider if you're feeling run down and exhausted.

CULPRIT NUMBER ONE: NOT ENOUGH SLEEP
I thought I'd knock this one off first because it is super common and tends to fly below the radar a bit, despite the fact that a

quarter of us have insomnia at any one time. Not getting enough sleep is a first-world problem that is becoming more common as the years go by. We know statistically we are sleeping less. There was an interesting study back in 1998 by the National Sleep Foundation, which found that the average woman between 30 and 60 only clocks around six hours and forty-one minutes of sleep a night on work nights. Anecdotally, that number has dropped since then. And even if you get more than that some nights, you still may not be enough sleep across the week. In another 2002 study, a whopping 63 per cent of women experienced some sort of insomnia at least twice a week.

## A CLOSER LOOK AT SLEEP

Have you ever stopped to think about what sleep is? It's actually a state of non arousal in the brain. Your brain has a whole heap of centres and neurons solely dedicated to keeping you awake and alert. When your brain is awake it is metabolically active, when asleep it is very inactive, uses very little glucose and takes a break in every way.

The sleep and arousal centres in your brain generally sit in balance with wakefulness and arousal, powered by the neurotransmitters: orexin, histamine, noradrenaline and serotonin, which beat off the sleep centres. At night the sleep centres, powered by the calming neurotransmitters GABA and galanin, take over.

The brain simply cannot function all the time at the high metabolic level required when you're awake. It gets worn out. So chronic sleep deprivation drives the metabolism of the brain down, impairing its general function. You can't think as clearly, you feel a bit fuzzy in your head, it's harder to pick up new concepts and your emotions get out of control. You will cry at the drop of a hat, take offense at silly little things and yell at the kids for no good reason.

What's going on in insomnia? Either the sleep system is too weak to shut down the wake system or the wake system is too strong so it overpowers the sleep system at night time as well. Either way there's a hyper-arousal system at play. Research has confirmed recently that this hyper-arousal is there around the clock in most insomniacs, making them feel awake and full of nervous tension during the day as well as starting at the ceiling at night. Sure they feel exhausted but they can't nap because even during the day their brains are spinning at twice normal speed making it impossible to shut down the arousal centres.

Many patients say they can't sleep because 'Doc, I can't shut my brain off. It just keeps going.' The obvious thought is 'Oh, you're stressed!' But we now know that's not the cause of the insomnia. It seems that instead they have an engine that's idling too high. And their overactive brains start thinking about stuff because that's what you do at one in the morning when you're lying in bed and have no one to chat with to get your mind off problems.

We know that the hypothalamus in someone who is an insomniac will release more CRH (corticotrophin releasing hormone – head back to the Hormone Primer for a refresher!) and as a result get a higher level of cortisol in the blood stream. Don't confuse this with the pseudoscientific concept of adrenal fatigue, which doesn't exist. I'm just saying that with all the negative things that come with excess cortisol in your blood stream, getting enough sleep can reverse many of them.

Getting enough sleep is vital. People with a sleep disorder are four hundred per cent more likely to develop depression than good sleepers.

Ok enough said! Get some sleep and see your doctor if you need help to do that.

## How to handle your tiredness

Above and beyond the specific advice I've given you above, I thought I'd give you some general energy boosters that will help nearly all of us with tiredness.

### DRINK UP

Water that is – not booze! So many of us walk around with nowhere near the requisite fluids on board. Women need to drink 2.1 litres of fluid per day on top of our food to stay well hydrated. That assumes you're not exercising more than a stroll around the block and you're neither pregnant nor breast-feeding. Think about it – it seriously is eight glasses of water per day.

There was a terrific study done in the USA where women in

various stages of hydration were measured for things like exercise tolerance, fatigue and concentration. I don't think anyone will have their socks blown off to find out that dehydrated women felt more tired and found everything from walking on a treadmill to sitting on a computer more difficult. Getting enough fluid can be hard, especially when you don't like water. As soft drinks are really a no-no, we will have to get creative.

I am going to share some of my tips as I am always battling to stay hydrated. I'm busy at work and as much as I love tea and coffee, I just don't have the time to put the kettle on and wait for it to boil. If it's not on my desk, it's not going to happen. So when I wake up I have a couple of cups of tea, a coffee or two and a glass of water. I multitask – so I drink while I'm getting the kids up and unstacking the dishwasher and that sort of thing. During the day I get a big water bottle that can last me the whole day. In it I like to have either some fresh mint leaves, a couple of slices of fresh ginger or a smashed cardamom pod. I know people who go for lemon or lime slices as well. Or you could make some herbal tea and let it go cold and shove that in a (non BPA) water bottle.

From the NH and MRC's perspective, fluid is fluid. They don't care whether it is juice, milk, soft drink or water, or a hot drink like tea or coffee – FROM A HYDRATION PERSPECTIVE. I do care though. I think soft drinks are diabolical. They're linked to strokes, heart disease and diabetes as well as obesity. There are so many added chemicals to soft drinks and yet absolutely NO nutritional value whatsoever is added. If you love the fizz, try sparkling water instead. If you are watching your weight then fruit juice is only a teency weency step up from soft drink. Juices really are loaded with kilojoules you don't need and don't even have the best fibrous parts of the fruit left in them. I know they're less processed and artificial but they're still calorie bombs.

### HAVE A LATTE

While you're drinking up, I have good news for you. Coffee not only counts towards your 2.1 litres a day of fluid, but it will give you a nice little health kick as well. A coffee is the way lots of us kick start our brains for the day. The caffeine and fluid together are great for boosting brain power. But don't see it as a vice. Apart from being a great source of antioxidants, coffee contains the world's favourite stimulant, caffeine. You will hear 'experts' like your mother-in-law or health food store salesperson advising you to detox off coffee pronto to boost your energy levels. Complete trollop. As I said, coffee is packed with antioxidants.

For a start, a recent US study found that men who drank two to three cups of coffee a day had a 10 per cent lower risk for dying during the 13 years of the study than men who drank no coffee. In that same study, women who drank two to three cups of coffee daily had a 13 per cent lower risk of death. It's not just me. Coffee is a life saver!

In addition, coffee drinkers seem to get less depression. In a study of more than 50,000 women, the ones who drank two to three cups of coffee per day had a 15 per cent decreased risk of depression than the ones who drank one cup or less of caffeinated coffee per week. And those who drank four cups of coffee per day or more had a 20 per cent lower risk.

Coffee also decreases the likelihood you will get diabetes. In a major review of several studies, it turned out that the more coffee people drink, the less their chances of going on to develop diabetes. For every extra cup of coffee drunk per day you get an extra seven per cent reduction in your risk of getting diabetes.

A Swedish study found that women who drank five cups of coffee per day significantly lowered their risk of developing breast cancer after the menopause.

Coffee also protects the liver, preventing scarring from weight gain and fatty liver disease. Coffee drinkers also get 25 per cent fewer strokes, less heart disease, less dementia and Parkinson's disease, lower insulin levels and less chance of gout. Studies also show drinking coffee (not swallowing caffeine tablets) helps overweight people lose weight.

Some people are more sensitive than others to caffeine and can feel their heart racing after just one cup. You can build up tolerance to the side effects of caffeine but some people are just never able to tolerate it. Lots of my patients with irritable bowel syndrome can't handle coffee either. As soon as they have a coffee, they're heading to the toilet with tummy cramps and a bit of diarrhea.

If you get either of those problems, you can try switching to decaf, which should fix the problem. The only problem is that most of the studies that have found the major health benefits from coffee haven't looked at decaf coffee. So while we think the health benefits from coffee come from the healthy anti-oxidants, they might also be helped along by caffeine. In this case, decaf won't be quite as healthy an option but it will give you some benefits. And at least it tastes good. Unless you really dislike coffee.

### MEDITATE

The fatigue-busting powers of meditation have been investigated and proven numerous times. But lots of people hear the word meditate and think cheesecloth kaftans and incense or people who are so chilled anyway that they practically meditate through life. I hear it all the time; "I've tried meditating and I can't do it!" I think that's because the concept of meditation is way too complex. It doesn't need to be full of Omms and Chakras and lotus positions. You can do a quick form of meditation that really, really works. Trust me, I'm a doctor. These are the steps to follow.

* Sit on a comfortable chair. Put your bottom right back in the chair. Make sure your feet are resting gently on the ground, equally weighted.
* Gently close your eyes, don't scrunch your eyelids up, just rest them very gently together.
* Relax your feet, resting them gently on the floor.
* Relax your thighs letting them fall into the chair.
* Let your tummy blob out, no holding it all in!
* Let your shoulders drop.
* Let your hands rest comfortably on your lap.
* Relax your brow.
* Unclench your jaw.
* Now take a long, slow breath in through your nose and out again, through your nose.
* As you breathe, focus all of your mind on the way the air feels cooler and sharper going in and warmer and softer going out.
* Just focus on the way the breath feels on the tip of your nose.
* If your mind wanders, imagine yourself gently scooping your thoughts back and placing them gently on the tip of your nose.

When it comes to meditating, it won't happen overnight, but it will happen. The secret is to practice. Start with 20 minutes a day. Once you are good at it and can switch your mind off quickly you can do it whenever you want and when you need it most. And you can add in a five-minute meditation when you're feeling exhausted if you can find a park bench or quiet spot to sit.

### Move it! Move it!

Do some exercise. Around 80 studies have all shown that your mental alertness improves both during and after exercise, regardless of the type of exercise. Even when you couldn't think of anything you feel like less, regular exercisers feel more energetic generally but moving your butt also gives you an instant kick! In a really old but absolutely classic study out of California State University, sugar hits were pitted against brisk walks in a mighty battle of the instant energy boosters. A 10 minute brisk walk trumped the sugar hit. A simple short walk gave the people in the study a good two hours of extra energy. The sugar hit gave an instant energy bounce, but an hour later energy levels had fallen even further than they were to begin with. So, 10 minutes! Think you could handle that?

### Get some sunshine

The sleep hormone melatonin is switched off by bright lights. Your first choice is sunshine. Did you know that even on a cloudy day sunlight is far brighter than TV studio lighting? A good dose of sunshine first thing in the morning will switch off your melatonin and give your brain a good wake up. You only need five minutes. If this is hard to do on a weekday morning when getting out the door to work is enough of a chore without adding another thing to your to-do list, try multi-tasking. Hang out your washing first thing if you can. Or go outside or onto a balcony to do your hair and make-up. Or at least try to open ALL your curtains and blinds to let the sunshine flood your home. If it is truly a horrid day or you wake up pre-dawn, switch on ALL your lights as artificial light is a good second best.

### Energy overhaul

Identify (and ditch) the energy sappers in your life. We all have at least one. Someone who, after spending five minutes talking to them, you want to go away and lie down. They're dripping with negativity. Everything is dreadful and nothing can fix it. You have to listen to their chat with its interminable detail and nothing up-beat you have to offer will penetrate their armour-plated misery. These people are energy murderers. Sorry if it's your mum or your best friend, but less contact is more if you're feeling ex-hausted.

# Are My Hormones Making Me Fat?

It's the sort of question I hear so frequently in my surgery. There's nothing that makes me feel like more of a dinosaur than realising that more and more of the things that I was taught at university are being debunked and former sacred cows are now completely old-school. Case in point – your weight. I remember being told that calories in greater than calories out was the road to overweight and obesity. For ages I've intrinsically known that's not right. I've had too many patients basically shattered by the fact that they are 'being good' – not perfect – but a whole heap better than their peers, yet are either not losing any weight at all, or their progress is so slow it's heartbreaking. Are hormones big players in weight gain? You bet!

## It's all in your genes

Ask anyone what determines how tall they grow and almost 100 per cent would agree it's their genes. For some reason we're more sceptical about the role genes play in determining our weight.

But from studies, it is estimated that around 60 per cent of our weight is determined by our genes.

There is a complex interplay between our lifestyle, how much exercise we do, how much and what we eat, and the genes preset in our body. Genes control our hunger levels, our taste for certain foods and...Yep! Our hormones!!

# The hormone players in weight gain

Sure we went through these back in our hormone primer, but these guys are so important that they are worth revisiting.

## Leptin – the appetite suppressor to end all appetite suppressors

A relative new kid on the block in terms of our scientific knowledge, leptin is a hormone that is produced in and released from fat cells. In the lab, if you take rats and basically inject leptin into their blood or directly into their brains (don't think about that too much!!) they drop their food intake and body weight. The more leptin you give the rats, the more marked their weight reduction. Leptin receptors have been found in lots of body organs, including the brain, especially in the hypothalamus, one of the parts of the brain at the forefront of controlling your appetite and food intake.

It also makes your cells more sensitive to insulin and so less insulin is needed to shift glucose into the cells. That would be a good thing for those of us trying to watch our weight.

The amount of leptin produced by both humans and rats is proportional to body fat. Just think about it; the fatter you get, the more leptin you make. So you should stop eating once you gain a bit of weight, right? Wrong. We know that. For a start when leptin was first discovered, scientists rushed to see whether leptin could be turned into a kind of obesity medicine – 'Here: take this and you won't want to eat any more!' It was a massive fail. Plus, we all know that one of the biggest issue people who carry too much weight around face is that they're really hungry lots of the time. It turns out that in humans, becoming obese makes you insensitive to leptin. It's in the blood telling you to STOP eating and that you're NOT hungry but you can't hear it.

Your brain has just stopped listening to its cues.

Well it turns out that in obese, diabetic mice, some also have an abnormality in their leptin receptors in the brain as well. So while these mice have tons of leptin in their blood streams, their brain receptors can't recognize it properly and so don't respond to it. In other mice, their receptors look normal but as they gain weight, they need much HIGHER levels of leptin to get switched on.

Mice and rats are scarily similar to us genetically and so we can assume that what happens in a mouse, happens in us and as we get bigger we develop leptin resistance. Whether they were born with leptin resistance which made them fat and diabetic or whether becoming fat made them leptin resistance is under investigation now. We're still not sure.

As an interesting aside, leptin seems to have a more complex role than simply regulating your appetite. It seems to be vital to hitting puberty and starting to regulate the female hormones as well and seems to contribute to the healthy development of the brain and immune system. It's early days and I'm sure we will hear more about this new discovery very soon.

## Ghrelin – the carb me up hormone

If you remember back to the Hormone Primer, ghrelin is your appetite turbo booster. Made in the stomach and pancreas, ghrelin is an appetite stimulant with receptors in the brain, especially the hypothalamus and pituitary gland and the whole gastrointestinal tract. In response to a burst of ghrelin from the stomach, you crave food. It also switches your pituitary gland on to make more growth hormone.

But beyond simply stimulating your appetite, ghrelin helps you build up some nice fat supplies by telling your tissues to grab calories and divert them into the fat cells. On the other hand it, ahem, gets you moving. A big dose of ghrelin switches on your guts and makes them 'move' things along a little faster.

What drives up your ghrelin? Well besides having an empty stomach and a pre-programmed meal time, lack of sleep is a major trigger to pump up the ghrelin levels. It seems that your brain needs sleep, but left without enough of its petrol of choice, it will tell your brain to drive you towards the cookie jar for a sugar hit by an extra hit of ghrelin. I'm sure you've noticed that on days when sleep is in short supply you feel hungrier? That'd be your hormones!

Ghrelin levels drop after gastric bypass surgery but increase after dieting, which may explain why diet-induced weight loss can be difficult to maintain. People with obesity and overweight have low ghrelin levels, probably because they're never starving enough for the levels to skyrocket. But there's another theory that goes that the ghrelin receptors in the brain of obese people are super sensitive, so that even with really low levels in the blood, they're still hungry all the time. Ghrelin doesn't just control feeding. Grehlin helps your brain to grow and adapt to changes. It is anti-inflammatory and helps with healing within the gastrointestinal tract.

## Insulin – the best and the worst

If you remember, insulin, sent into the bloodstream by the islet cells of your pancreas is responsible for allowing glucose, the main sugar which is your cells' main fuel into the cells. Glucose cannot get into the heart of the cell unless insulin unlocks the door of the cell. Remember that insulin is the key, and your insulin receptors are the locks on the doors of your cells. Your pancreas pushes out more insulin when the pancreas detects a decent blood sugar amount which signals the need for a little help to get the sugar from the blood into the cells where it's needed, but also just from the sight and taste of food.

Insulin is good stuff to have in a famine. It assumes you may not see another decent meal for many a day and helps you conserve every single kilojoule your body encounters and store it for a rainy, food-free day.

More sugar in the blood than you need? No worries! Insulin ensures it gets packed away in the liver as the sugar storage molecule, glycogen. Once the liver's glycogen storage units are full to capacity, insulin is on the job, telling your liver to make fat out of the incoming sugars. These storage fats are then packed off and sent out into the blood stream to be stored in offsite storage facilities (like your butt, thighs and round your middle).

Plus for good measure, it triggers the fat cells themselves to make its own fat for storage out of any excess sugar it finds. The last thing insulin does is to turn off fat burning.

But, if you think all insulin does is turn you into a metabolic fat-making machine, there's more! If you were faced with a rare meal in a time of famine, feeling full and not being able to eat the meal in front of you would be dangerous, right? So insulin is on the job with its very own over-ride switch in your brain, switching off the 'I'm full' signals and tricking you into feeling hungry, even when you aren't. Even when you've eaten so much, you're really, really full! People with high insulin levels (see below) feel hungrier, crave more sugar, enjoy sweet things more and, no surprise, eat more than people with lower insulin levels. If you've ever felt starving half an hour after dinner, even though you've eaten so much your pants are tight, chances are you have a tad too much insulin on board.

# Are my hormones making me fat?

In medicine we often look at 'case studies' to examine a medical problem. So Let me give you a case study now drawn from the hundreds of women I see in this predicament who do indeed have hormonal weight gain and have felt like a fat failure until getting the correct diagnosis (which can take years if not decades).

### KELLY
Kelly came to see me at 26 years of age with some bleeding on the pill. It didn't take long for her to tell me she was worried about her weight.

About three months ago she was absolutely sick of herself and her bulges, especially around the middle. She was about to be a bridesmaid for her cousin and really wanted to shed a few (more than a few) kilos before the wedding. She had acknowledged that while her whole life had been spent dieting, and her weight yo-yo-ing up and down, she'd never really given it 100 per cent. So now she was getting serious. She had enrolled with a personal trainer at huge expense and he had given her a diet to follow. But four months later she had only shed 500 grams despite working her butt off and basically obsessing over her meals, measuring out grams of rice and tuna. She felt hopeless and miserable.

She'd been to see doctors before. They'd do blood tests and tell her that everything was fine including her thyroid hormones and her sugar levels. She felt they just thought she was lying about what she ate and that she was just a pathetic chocoholic with no sense of self control. Ironically, she said that's what she had been all her life, but this time she wasn't.

We took a look back at Kelly's hormonal life. When she'd started her periods they were absolutely all over the show and very, very painful. She missed school a few days from period pain. At 16 her mum had finally let her go on the pill to sort out her periods and they'd settled down nicely. But she'd started to put on weight. She was a fairly sedentary teenager and didn't do much sport, and ate her share of junk food, but no more than her friends, and yet she was much chubbier than many of them. She also had acne and she had developed some embarrassing hairs on her snail trail (on the tummy) and around the nipples. She was too embarrassed to ask any of her friends about it but assumed that was all normal and just plucked them out.

She always suffered from pretty bad mood swings as a teenager and her mum called her 'hormonal'. In reality she just hated her appearance. She felt fat, ugly and hairy. As she got older the weight was a constant battle. She had tried shakes, a dietician, the Zone diet, the Atkins diet, Weight Watchers, every celebrity diet published in a magazine; she had spent her entire salary on weight loss supplements. Everything would work a BIT for a time, but she would always bounce back and then some. Her lack of success in weight loss made her even more miserable.

Now with her job as a personal assistant she was pretty sedentary and sat most of the day. Come 3 or 4 pm she would find it hard to concentrate, feel light-headed, sometimes shaky, often cranky and would CRAVE sugar like a madwoman. Only recently had she shaken the overpowering urge to head to the tea room for a cream-filled-biscuit to right her sugar levels.

She'd also recently gone off the pill to 'give her body a break' but the periods had become erratic again and after tolerating that roller coaster for a year, she'd gone to a medical centre for another script to whip her hormones back into line. DOES THIS SOUND LIKE YOU?

This story could make me weep every time I hear it. The years of self loathing, the failed attempts to right the weight wrongs. The guilty eating, the dieting, the feeling that nothing will work anyway. And most of all, the absolute dismal failure by doctors to get what this is and fix it. The lack of compassion for what is a soul-destroying experience.

We did a series of blood tests on Kelly to confirm what I suspected already – she had polycystic ovarian syndrome together with insulin resistance (terms I will explain in a minute) and she DEFINITELY had hormonal weight gain.

## Hormonal weight gain

If you have struggled with diet after diet, done spin class after power walk, gone for shakes, tried supplements and joined torturous programs involving meetings that could make you cry from boredom... and still hardly lost any weight, chances are you have a hormonal imbalance. And in the case of polycystic ovarian syndrome AKA PCOS, that's exactly what you've got – a hormonal imbalance.

## Is my Polycystic Ovary Syndrome (PCOS) making me fat?

Between eight and ten percent of women in that fertile age bracket between the time of getting your periods and menopause have PCOS. The hormonal imbalances are across the board. The hormones that control ovulation don't work properly and as a result you develop cysts all over the ovaries (see below). You end up with a cascade of hormonal issues with the net result being that you don't ovulate properly so your cycle goes haywire and instead of the nice cycling of oestrogen and progesterone we met in the Hormone primer, your ovaries and adrenals make an excess of male hormones with a whole raft of side effects. Lastly, it usually (but not always) comes packaged up with insulin resistance.

Your cells need a couple of forms of petrol to power them. Oxygen makes its own merry way into the cell without any help from any hormones. As you now know very well, sugar, on the other hand, can't go it alone. Insulin is like the key that unlocks the doors to allow sugar into your cells. In insulin resistance the insulin is there aplenty (unlike Type I Diabetes where the pancreas fails to produce enough) but the locks on the cell doors have gone a bit rusty and aren't working as efficiently. As a result, the control of your sugar levels in your cells and the amount of sugar in your blood goes awry. Sometimes the system works well, other times there is a sugar queue building up in the blood stream with a net deficit inside the cells where it is needed.

Unfortunately with insulin resistance, the body doesn't work out that this is simply a matter of needing some grease on the insulin receptor locks. As far as your pancreas is concerned, a sugar build up in the blood means one thing and one thing only; pump out more insulin. As we now know, insulin is a brilliant STORAGE hormone – the storage in this case is FAT. Excess insulin means your body will scavenge every calorie in your body to turn into fat and will halt fat burning.

As far as your pancreas is concerned, a sugar build-up in the blood means one thing and one thing only; pump out more insulin. As we now know, insulin is a brilliant storage hormone and in this case it stores fat. Excess insulin means your body will scavenge every calorie in your body to turn into fat and will halt fat burning.

How do you know you have the PCOS, insulin resistance or both? The telltale signs (and you can have all or just some) are:

* Erratic, irregular cycles (usually your periods come less frequently rather than more because you are ovulating less often).

* Hairiness in places you don't like such as around the nipples, on the tummy, the face or back (because your androgen or male hormone levels are too high) See Are My Hormones Making Me Look Bad?

* Your hair on your head is thinning and falling out or receding (same thing – androgen overload)

* You develop acne often in dodgy spots like your back and chest as well as your face (androgen overload as well), See Are My Hormones Making Me Look Bad?

* Difficulty shifting weight and a tendency to pack it on easily (this is because you often have higher insulin levels due to insulin resistance – see below)

* Moodiness or stress. Fifty per cent of women with PCOS

do suffer mood disturbance as well – see Are My Hormones Making Me Moody?

* Infertility (because the hormones stop eggs being released from the ovaries properly)
* Skin issues – include pigmentation of the skin on the knuckles and toes (this usually fades after 40 years), pigmentation under the eyes and on the eyelids and in the armpits and neck and lots of skin tags.
* Family history. If either of your parents has diabetes or insulin resistance or ever had polycystic ovaries or diabetes of pregnancy, your genes could be affected.
* Tiredness. Exhaustion. (Your sugar isn't moving into the cells adequately leaving you tired and worn out.) See Are My Hormones Making Me Tired?

## What causes PCOS and IR?

Consider this whole topic a work in progress as we're still discovering more and more about this condition all the time. Like nearly everything in your body, the starting point is your genes. You're born with them courtesy of your parents and they inhabit the nucleus or core of every cell in your body. The genes for this condition are probably incredibly advantageous in a famine. Because having lots of insulin means you would be able to survive longer without food. But in our times of plenty, they are pretty devastating. Not all of the genes for this condition have yet been identified, and the chances are there are a whole raft of them and it's likely that the worse the combination and the greater the number of these genes, the worse the condition is.

Dodgy genes can be activated by a bad environment and in my experience, your body doesn't need a massive hammering to do just that. Lots of us at 17, 18 or even in our early 20s went through a phase of eating junk (because we could and didn't put on weight), drinking too much and dropping out of exercise altogether. These days we're seeing it happen early in childhood. But if you have those dodgy PCOS and insulin resistance genes, this sort of lifestyle mess can activate your genes and create havoc with your hormones.

And remember that corticotrophin-releasing hormone or CRH

(again back to the Hormone Primer) also switches off, or at least down, the important gonadotrophin-releasing hormone or GnRH. Now, as you will already know from the hormone primer, GnRH is responsible for the release of the important pituitary hormones, FSH and LH, which control the whole menstrual cycle. So stress can definitely stuff up your cycle as any stressed-out woman can tell you.

Once activated, it can be very difficult to switch your PCOS and insulin resistance genes off and once diagnosed with it, you should see PCOS and insulin resistance as lifelong conditions. Not that you have no hope of losing weight and clearing your skin. Far from it. The prognosis when treated properly is great. But you will have to be well managed for the rest of your life.

## How PCOS stuffs up your monthly (or hormonal) cycle

Remember back to the Hormone Primer when we were describing how the whole menstrual cycle basically works? Luteinizing hormone or LH stimulates the follicles to release an egg. Well, in a normal cycle, follicles only respond to that LH surge when they have matured to a diameter of nine mm or more. But that system is disrupted in PCOS and insulin resistance. Excess insulin in the blood makes smaller, immature follicles as small as four mm sensitive to your LH so that they respond prematurely to LH but aren't yet ready to release an egg or form a decent corpus luteum. In addition, your high insulin levels also stimulate your pituitary to pump out higher levels of LH as well. So between your high LH and these hypersensitive follicles, ovulation doesn't happen properly and you have all of these overstimulated follicles.

OK now, once again, here I'm going to go all science nerd on you and revisit the menstrual cycle again. But bear with me because it is worth understanding. The follicles are the groups of cells which house and then release an egg AND produce hormones. Each month seemingly randomly an egg is CHOSEN and it then wakes up the surrounding ovary cells known as the 'primordial follicle' to become proper mature FOLLICLES. One important cell type which basically sits in a layer around the outside of the follicle is the layer of theca cells. They form a kind of fence or netting that holds the follicle together, but that's not all.

When stimulated by that pituitary hormone LH, the theca cells produce the androgen called androstenedione which the neighbouring 'granulosa cells' on the inside of the follicle need to make oestrogen through the enzyme aromatase that we met in The Hormone Primer. Remember this? Normally, after ovulation, the egg is released, the rest of the follicle's cells die off but the theca cells then transform into basically their own little hormone powerhouse called the corpus luteum. This unit makes tonnes of progesterone. Still with me?

In PCOS the theca cells just keep growing but the granulosa cells often suffer a premature death and you end up with lots of half baked follicles without eggs in them. They look like tiny little cysts.

Let's deal first with that overgrowth of theca cells, which causes too much androstenedione to be produced and then with less granulosa cells around, all that androsteniodione simply can't be converted to oestrogen. Instead much will be converted to testosterone by the theca cells themselves. The result is lots of androgens in your system and as a result your hair growth goes ballistic everywhere you don't want it, you can lose the stuff on your head and your face (and back) and get covered with zits to a greater or lesser degree. The extent to which this happens is dependent on how severe your PCOS is and also your genes which determine the location, number and sensitivity of your androgen receptors. Meanwhile, back to the insulin; it stimulates the adrenal glands which sit like little hats on top of the kidneys to produce even more androgens.

The lack of progesterone because of the failure to ovulate leaves your body in an oestrogen dominant state. One problem is that with only oestrogen circulating, the endometrium builds up with lots of rich blood but without progesterone to pack it down and organise it, it gets too bulky. That means periods are often longer and heavier, sometimes with clots.

I will deal with acne, hairiness (hirsutism) and hair loss from your head in the final chapter (Are My Hormones Making Me Look Bad?)

## Long-term effects of PCOS

Many women with PCOS put lots of focus on their weight issues, their skin or maybe their infertility. But from my perspective as a doctor, I'm also worried about the long-term health effects of this condition. Women with PCOS have a seven-fold increased risk of type two diabetes mellitus. They also have a much higher risk of vascular diseases that lead to stroke and heart attack. In fact by age 19, women with PCOS already have thickened artery linings compared with women without this problem.

Then there's the relatively rare endometrial cancer or cancer of the lining of the uterus. Women with PCOS have a fourfold increase of this endometrial carcinoma compared to women without. That's a result of the imbalance between oestrogen and progesterone levels that again happens because the ovarian follicles just simply don't work properly. Plus insulin is a cancer promoter all on its own. Insulin receptors are numerous on the surfaces of cancer cells in diabetics.

What often devastates my patients most is the sub fertility and high miscarriage rate of PCOS. We see huge benefits in both from aggressively treating the condition, but those issues are often the impetus to take the disease seriously and pull out all stops to get it under control.

## Insulin resistance

What lots of my patients come in to discuss is the fact that they've dieted to hell and back and after two weeks of back- breaking work at the gym and living on what feels like a carrot and two lettuce leaves a day, they've lost a grand total of 200 grams and feel absolutely heartbroken. It is so hard to keep going, being so diligent, and working so hard for what feels like no reward. It's no wonder so many women in this situation throw in the towel and give up.

That's where we do the fasting blood tests which so often reveal that what is going on for these people is a case of hormonal weight gain – also known as insulin resistance. In insulin resistance there is plenty of insulin around but it isn't working that well inside the body. To revisit the analogy I used earlier, insulin is the key that unlocks the doors of the cells to allow sugar in. In insulin resistance the insulin receptors on the cells, or 'the locks', get rusty and don't work that well. As a result, the sugar can't get out of the blood stream into the cells where it is needed and your body responds to the high level of sugar in the blood by pumping out more insulin.

As you will remember from the Hormone Primer, insulin is a powerful inhibitor of fat burning (lipolysis). Just to put some numbers around this, after a meal, if you are healthy, the highest insulin level we see is around 40 micrograms per litre. Now we know that your body simply cannot break down fat until your insulin falls to a level of around eight micrograms per litre or below. In healthy people, this happens around two or two and half hours after a meal. If you have insulin resistance, realistically you may never drop your insulin to levels low enough to allow fat to break down. In fact many of my patients who have a simple fasting insulin level done through a blood test find it NEVER falls below around 14 or 15 micrograms per litre. I've seen fasting insulin levels above 100. As you can imagine, it is no wonder that these people report finding it impossible to lose weight even when they protest, "I'm being so good!" Meanwhile, remembering back to what insulin does for your body, with insulin levels that high, your body is going to be on a scavenger hunt for every single stray calorie to pack away as storage fat. Insulin makes that process so easy, meaning you put ON weight at the drop of a hat.

In insulin resistance, the enlarged fat cells behave differently to normal fat cells. They produce two hormones called TNF-*a* and resistin which make your muscles more insulin resistant. Now the whole cycle gets worse, because the more insulin resistant your cells are, the worse your body's ability to handle carbohydrates and once again, all that sugar hanging around in the blood makes your pancreas produce more insulin and the cycle keeps getting worse.

Brain PET scans of people with and without insulin resistance has shown that the usual response of the brain to switch off the hunger centre in the hypothalamus of the brain after a meal doesn't work in people with insulin resistance. Which means in spite of having enough calories on board, they will still seek more food. Plus insulin makes you crave sugary foods and you really enjoy sweet foods more than people with normal insulin levels.

All in all, insulin resistance is like a runaway train to weight gain and no wonder people diagnosed with the disorder have a 50 per cent chance of developing type II Diabetes within 10 years of the diagnosis unless treated properly.

When I tell my patients whose blood tests come back revealing insulin resistance they have hormonal weight gain, so many of them don't know whether to laugh or cry. First comes the enormous relief that there's a REASON why this is happening. There's a medical explanation for their weight gain. They're not just being a hopeless sloth with no self control. They're not imagining it.

That's quickly followed by the realisation that this condition is something they are going to have to overcome in order to lose weight, get their looks sorted, improve their mood (see Are My Hormones Making Me Moody?) And the reality of what lies ahead is daunting. They must face a future either without the foods they love and crave or with them but paying a heavy (literally) toll for each sugary snack that they consume.

## Diagnosing PCOS and insulin resistance

Diagnosing these conditions can be hard. The clinical story is enough to raise our suspicions and any blood testing is only used to confirm the diagnosis and benchmark where you're at. There are problems with most of the tests as you will see.

### PELVIC ULTRASOUND

We're looking for the telltale cysts on the ovaries. There don't need to be that many of them to get a pair of ovaries that 'could be consistent with PCOS in the right clinical setting'. In other words, it is not enough to conclude you have PCOS simply on the basis of an ultrasound alone but it helps to build the picture of what's happening inside your body. Beware, though, that over 20 per cent of "normal" women have polycystic ovaries on ultrasound. And only 75 per cent of women with PCOS have polycystic ovaries on ultrasound, so it is not a perfect test by any means.

### ORAL GLUCOSE TOLERANCE TEST (OGTT) WITH INSULIN

This test is a series of blood glucose tests. You fast overnight, then turn up at the lab and get a fasting glucose and insulin level done. Then you are given a very sweet sugary drink which is designed to "challenge" your carbohydrate metabolic system. You have another set of glucose and insulin tests an hour later and then another hour after that. You can't run around between tests as this can artificially elevate your sugar level. So come with a book and be prepared to hang around for a couple of hours. We usually suggest you eat a diet with lots of carbs in the three days before the test. If you're on a low carb or no carb diet, you can get a 'false negative' test result.

### HORMONE TESTS

There is no point in doing hormone tests if you're on the pill as they all get distorted so we only do these tests if you're not on the pill:

* Androgens. This includes 'free androgen index' (the free unbound proportion of male hormone in your blood), and can sometimes include DHEAS (might be normal or slightly elevated) or androstenedione levels (see the hormone primer) to detect high circulating androgens

* SHBG Sex-hormone-binding globulin (SHBG) is a protein that binds to both testosterone and oestradiol. If the SHBG is low the amount of active testosterone can skyrocket. Therefore, it is very important to measure SHBG in all patients being evaluated for polycystic ovarian syndrome. You should never measure androgens without SHBG.

* LH:FSH ratio This is sometimes done. A ratio ≥2.0 LH:FSH is suggestive of PCOS but is not very accurate.

### THYROID HORMONE TESTS

Studies suggest that women with PCOS may be four times more likely to suffer from an underactive thyroid due to Hashimoto's thyroiditis, an autoimmune disease of the thyroid gland. (See Are My Hormones Making Me Tired?) We think that the imbalance between oestrogen and progesterone affects your immune system, making immune problems of the thyroid gland more common. Plus an underactive thyroid can make your PCOS worse because it can lower your SHBG (sex hormone binding globulin) which in turn can lead to higher concentrations of free testosterone. I ALWAYS screen for an underactive thyroid when I'm investigating Insulin resistance and PCOS.

### Vitamin D level

Studies have found that up to 75 per cent of women with PCOS have low vitamin D levels. Vitamin D is activated in the skin by sunlight. It is harder to find in food. While we don't know for sure that low vitamin D CAUSES or WORSENS PCOS and IR, there is a strong link. So if we do find vitamin D deficiency we will always correct it.

### 24-hour urine-free cortisol

This is sometimes done. You collect all the urine you do in a 24-hour period (yup that is a LOT) and the total amount of cortisol (the stress hormone) is measured. Mildly elevated levels can be seen in PCOS with values more than double the upper limit of normal. It gives us an indication of the extent to which stress is playing a role in your condition.

But remember, these tests are important but the diagnosis is going to rest more with the history you give and your appearance. Having diagnosed this condition, we have to manage it.

## How to handle your hormones

Here is the hard reality; insulin resistance is partly due to your genes being activated and so you will not CURE it but instead will MANAGE it, eliminating the symptoms and prevent long-term consequences.

The three pillars of treatment are
* Exercise
* Weight loss
* Medications that improve insulin sensitivity

You also need to pay attention to things in your life that exacerbate the problem like work or relationship stress, mood disturbance or hormonal contraception.

Let's look further at the three pillars:

## EXERCISE

Exercise is THE MOST IMPORTANT part of managing PCOS and IR. All the experts I speak to agree that without exercise, it will be very difficult to get on top of this condition. Exercise actually sensitizes the muscles' insulin receptors to insulin meaning your body can lower its insulin levels and wind back some of the diabolical effects of high insulin on fat cells, the ovaries, your mind etc.

I absolutely promise you that even if you are not losing weight (and if you can't work out why that is the case go back to the beginning and try to remember the enormous hormonal hurdles you're trying to jump over here), you are still bumping up your insulin sensitivity. That has enormous benefits for your mood, the way you concentrate, your cycle and your skin. Even smaller amounts of exercise will do this so while more is more, even a little will help.

Now if you want to lose weight from exercise, unless you're an exercise lover, the news isn't going to make you smile. Unfortunately, the whole rule about 30 minutes a day five days a week for good overall health will leave you way short of the mark with hormonal weight gain. When your insulin levels are high, to bring them down, you'll need to do lots of exercise. Studies show that women with insulin resistance who exercise for 45–60 minutes, five to seven days a week, can lower their insulin levels, particularly peak levels, into the normal range and start to lose weight. Less than that and you might struggle a bit unless you're really excellent with your diet (see below). Of course that is completely unrealistic for most women. Plus every little bit counts. But the bottom line is that you really have to do AS MUCH EXERCISE AS YOU CAN and see it as part of the three pillars, rather than the single answer.

The key to picking up exercise is to find a way to not hate it. I can bang on about exercise till the cows come home but if I advise running to a committed non runner, we're not going to get anywhere. You have to enjoy it (at least a little bit). So whether it's joining a group so it's a social activity, whether it's walking with a girlfriend at night after work, whether it's a work-out DVD in your own home, make sure it's something you don't detest because you're going to have to get married to it!

## AEROBIC EXERCISE (CARDIO)

I know we all hate this but you do need to get your heart rate up and sweat a bit to achieve the best effects of exercise. To calculate your heart rate you take your pulse by placing your index and third fingers on your neck just to the side of your windpipe to locate your carotid artery pulse. Do this for 15 seconds by the clock and multiply that number by four to calculate the number of heart beats per minute. When doing some decent moderate exercise, aim for 60 to 80 per cent of maximum predicted heart rate. Are you going cross-eyed from all the maths yet? Your maximum heart rate is calculated by subtracting your age from 220. So, if you're 40 years old, subtract 40 from 220, to get a maximum heart rate of 180, which is the maximum number of times your heart should beat per one minute while you're exercising.

So here's an example. You are 40 years old. Your maximum predicted heart rate is 220 – 40 = 180. 60 per cent of 180 = 108. 80 per cent of 180 = 144. So aim to get your heart rate up to somewhere between 108 and 144 beats per minute.

Remember that's your GOAL, not the starting point. Couch potatoes shouldn't try to start here. Getting your heart rate up that high isn't that easy for people who never do any exercise. So if you're just getting started into exercise, focus instead on the amount and the rigour of the exercise you undertake. Start by walking for five minutes a day, and each day increase the length and pace you walk at. You want to be a bit sweaty, breathing hard but not uncomfortable.

Ultimately walking won't be enough. I find it is hard to raise the heart rate by a long walk. It's lovely, but it will never get your heart pumping to the levels we need. Try adding in stairs, hills, carrying hand weights (see below) or building up to a slow jog then easing back a bit.

## RESISTANCE TRAINING

By resistance training, I mean any exercise where each effort is performed against a specific opposing force generated by resistance. That's a terribly technical definition but let me give you an example. In a push-up you are pushing the weight of your body up against gravity, which stresses (and strengthens) your arms and some of your back muscles. In a lunge you hold your body up putting stress on your quadriceps muscles.

Studies have repeatedly shown that doing resistance training increases your muscles' insulin sensitivity even if that means cutting back a bit on the time you have for aerobic exercise.

You don't need a personal trainer or expensive Pilates equipment to do resistance training. Here are some things you can do at home.

* Add weights to your walk. If the idea of walking around with massive hand weights makes you scream with embarrassment (hey! I agree!) You can buy these pretty cool arm weights now that look like bracelets (but don't feel like that!) and nobody will give you a second look if you stick them on your arms while you're walking.

* If you need a push to do your traditional resistance exercises including push-ups, lunges, and sit-ups, grab your kids! Kids LOVE doing these exercises so why not encourage them to do it with you? No, doing push-ups won't hurt or damage their little muscles or joints either.

* Normal hand weights are pretty cheap and you can do sets of various arm workouts in the privacy of your own home.

* Pelvic floor muscle exercises are sadly neglected by most of us until we go through the menopause and try to play mad catch up with our leakage issues! Doing ten minutes of pelvic floor exercises at work counts! I'm serious. You can even do those exercises while driving the kids to school or at work at your desk.

I have suggested to some of my patients that they search Youtube for a good resistance work out for some good ideas.

### Core strength

Trainer, Rachel Livingstone, who specialises in creating an evidence based workout for women with PCOS and insulin resistance told me that building core strength is essential for women with these conditions. As she explained: "it makes you do your cardio and resistance better".

Try pelvic floor exercises (a must for most women), abdominal crunches, the plank and bridges. I could describe these to you, but I do think it's a good investment to either get a single session with a personal trainer (preferably well trained) or attend a class to make sure you are doing the exercises properly and not putting unnecessary strain through the lower back or neck.

I'll put a word in here for yoga and pilates, both of which give you such a great core workout but are also fun and have clear benefits for so many medical conditions especially musculoskeletal conditions. Annette Rich, the physiotherapist I refer to, always sees better results when she is working on shoulder, knee or back injuries when pilates is added in to the physiotherapy regimen. Again, it is important to have a properly qualified instructor to ensure these exercises are done effectively and safely.

# Your diet

I refer to two fantastic nutritionists who get hormonal weight gain and tailor a diet to the needs of the patients. If you have access to this sort of nutritionist, then I urge you to go at least twice to get some help. It will be the best investment you ever made. BUT get a referral. Not all nutritionists work in this space and some of my patients have reported receiving the most BIZARRE advice. So IF you aren't sure or can't find someone who understands IR and hormonal weight gain, here are my top tips for tackling the problem form a dietary perspective:

### A LOW GI DIET

Some carbohydrates are broken down more quickly, releasing their sugars into the blood stream more quickly than others. The Glycaemic Index or GI tells you how quickly it will release the sugar from that carb and so how it will affect your blood sugar and insulin levels. In short, the lower a food's glycaemic index, the slower its release of sugars and the less likely it is to give you a blood sugar and insulin spike. In other words, the lower the GI, the better. Low GI foods are foods with a GI of 55 or less. High GI foods, with a GI of 70 or more will give you a rapid rise in sugar and then a sugar crash.

Many low-GI foods are high in fibre. Fibre rich foods are harder to digest so they stay in the gastrointestinal tract longer. They therefore give you higher and longer release of all the gut peptides we met in the Hormone Primer such as cholecystokinin, leptin and glucagons, all of which keep you fuller for longer.

You can find out the GI of most foods from a good nutritionist or nutritional counsellor.

Examples include switching from a processed cereal like Corn Flakes to a traditional porridge or bran based cereal. Switch from white bread and rice crackers to wholegrain breads and high-fibre rye crackers. Switch from jasmine or short grain rice to basmati rice.

Similarly, some fruits are low GI while others are high GI. Apples, blueberries, strawberry, kiwi-fruit, oranges, rockmelons and peaches are fabulous low GI fruits. Bananas, nectarines, mangoes and watermelon are high GI.

### EMBRACE HUNGER

We know that if you have insulin resistance, your brain doesn't function properly to manage your appetite. We have found that your brain simply will not register that your calorie intake is adequate and switch on the appetite breaks. So to stop feeling hungry you'll have to wait until your stomach is so full that you can't fit any more in. That means inevitably that you will always overeat and that you will always feel hungrier than your buddies without IR.

So if you want to lose weight you have to accept that YOU WILL FEEL HUNGRY and that you can't listen to your brain's signals because they're dodgy. Don't worry that if you don't eat you'll pass out, you won't. You will feel cranky, moody, have a growling tummy, maybe be a little light-headed and even obsess about food but that will be the worst of it.

This too will pass. As your hormones begin to regulate and your stomach readjusts its hunger cues and the low GI food you're eating (see above) makes your sugar levels more regular thus avoiding the swinging pendulum of sugar cravings, low and high sugar levels.... You will feel better and you won't feel as hungry any more. I promise. Give it a month. Come on! You can do anything for a month right?

### SMALLER PORTION SIZES

Because you feel hungry all the time, many women with IR (and men too) overeat at every meal. Given that you have now told yourself that you're not really hungry, try to make your portion sizes smaller dictated by what is a reasonable meal size, not your appetite. I suggest plating your food in the kitchen and bringing it to the table.

You won't have a second helping because you will commit before starting to just finish what is on your plate.

### EAT REGULARLY

Women with PCOS and IR need to keep a stable sugar level to keep insulin levels as low as possible. As a result, if you have either or both of these conditions you should eat a small breakfast, lunch and dinner as well as two small snacks per day. There should be some protein as well as some low GI carb in each one of these small meals or snacks. Never ever skip meals.

### DON'T STARVE YOURSELF

I often see patients so determined to shift some weight that they start skipping meals thinking that less calories must be better for weight loss. Initially, with starvation we do see a drop in weight but it always rebounds quickly. For a start starving is unsustainable so you end up falling in a heap pretty quickly. Secondly your brain doesn't function that well in starvation mode and while you're trying to lose weight, you're also trying to sustain your relationships and cope at work so it's just not a good idea.

### DON'T OBSESS

While researching for this book I spoke to a nutritional counsellor called Ginette Lenham who specializes in IR and PCOS. She got into this field because she worked with people who had eating disorders and was horrified by the crossover between the two issues. It is so easy to understand how being dismissed by doctors, having low self-esteem because of your weight and looks, having a tendency to stress and be moody because of PCOS and IR, could combine to make you obsessive about food. Nearly everybody with these problems has dieted. It never works, making them get more and more extreme.

Ginette told me that women usually need to be told to RELAX more about their food. Stop weighing yourself (see below), don't measure out 100 grams of rice or tuna, stop daily pimple inspections. Be aware of the link between eating disorders and IR and PCOS and watch for signs that you are becoming a food obsessor and get help EARLY.

### EAT SLOWLY

One way to handle your appetite is to slow down the pace at which you eat. Didn't your mum and nanna always tell you to chew slowly? They were probably worried about you choking! But by eating slowly, you give your I'm Full hormones a better chance to reign in your appetite. Put your knife and fork down between each mouthful. Swallow and have a sip of water before taking the next mouthful. This will help you to eat less.

### DRINK WATER

Studies have shown that having a glass or two of water before a meal helps to trick your stomach into believing its full before you've overeaten your meal. It won't hurt and might help you reduce your portion sizes.

### DON'T BEAT YOURSELF UP

It is amazing that when it comes to weight loss, the self loathing and guilt that come with it can be the worst obstacles to success. You know what happens; you have a great plan. Right! This is it! Today I am really going to stick to my diet and exercise regime. I'm going to say no to cake at tea time! I'm going to buy a juicer and make carrot and parsley juice for an afternoon snack!!! I'm pumped! Until you slip up, as we all do. Usually once you've opened the pack of jelly beans, they're open right? And one thing leads to another and there goes one entire pack of jelly beans! Then comes the flood of guilt and self castigation. I'm so pathetic! I can't even last a day! No wonder I look like a fat pig! No wonder I don't have any decent clothes that fit me! What's the point??!! I can't do it! You can. Pull yourself off the floor, dust yourself off and the next hour is a new hour and you start again. Each fall off the horse, and there will be many, is a blip on your path to a slimmer, healthier, clear-skinned, fertile you!!

### FISH OIL SUPPLEMENT

The data here is a little thin. However, I do recommend either two 1000 mg fish oil tablets or two krill oil or other supplement containing the vital omega three fats, EPA and DHA. These are anti-inflammatory supplements and we know that women with PCOS and IR often have high levels of 'inflammatory markers' in their blood. Plus the results of small studies in humans and studies in rodents look promising. It's hard to know exactly what to make of the results as I never start a woman on a fish oil supplement without addressing the three pillars of exercise, diet and medication first and the general improvement we see can be hard to attribute to one particular change.

By the way if you're thinking that flax seed is a good alternative because you've read that on the internet, think again. Flax seed is indeed high in the fat, ALA which is normally converted to EPA and DHA. However if you do have insulin resistance, that conversion process tends to be less efficient, so you're better off sticking to the fish or krill oil.

## Medications for hormonal weight gain

While my advice is absolutely ALWAYS to see a fantastic nutritionist who GETS hormonal weight gain AND will work with you to understand your lifestyle to make your new diet work within your limits, the reality is that very often medication is required to get on top of the problem.

Now you might think that medication (which is called Metformin) is a way out of what is a pretty rigorous diet and exercise program, but it's not. It certainly really, really helps the diet and exercise move your weight loss along but sits with it, not instead of it. Studies consistently show that on its own, Metformin is a fail. Am I clear? If you eat a poor diet and go on Metformin, you will feel sick and not lose any weight. It is better to wait until you're ready to do this properly and then go for broke.

### METFORMIN

Metformin is an 'insulin-sensitising' medication that was invented to treat diabetes in 1957, but has been used to treat PCOS and IR since 1994. That was fairly experimental but studies in 2002 confirmed its role as a vital part of the management of this condition.

Metformin decreases the amount of sugar absorbed by the guts and makes the liver and muscles respond better to insulin by sensitising the receptors. It's really like greasing the rusty locks on your cells making the insulin key work better. This allows your body to achieve normal blood glucose levels with lower levels of insulin and that has a whole raft of effects including allowing fat burning, lowering your appetite, and less building of fat in the cells.

Metformin has been shown to rapidly improve fertility. For example in women with PCOS, 63 per cent of women will ovulate when they start Metformin compared to 67 per cent of women who start the ovulation stimulator, clomiphene citrate. Plus pregnancy rates are better, with 69 per cent of women with PCOS getting pregnant on Metformin compared to 34 per cent on clomiphene. Metformin also prevents miscarriages and all of this without the risk of a low blood sugar attack.

I find that slowly, slowly doctors are catching onto the usefulness of screening for PCOS and insulin resistance and of using Metformin. But often they use doses that are too small to achieve a significant movement in terms of weight, acne and cycle control. It is best taken twice or even three times a day to achieve optimum insulin control and we slowly increase the dose to achieve the best results.

Metformin is best taken WITH your meal. I advise my patients to take it with the first mouthful of breakfast and dinner.

The most common side effects of Metformin are:
* Nausea
* Loss of appetite
* Diarrhoea
* Increased abdominal gas

These side effects affect between 20 to 30 per cent of people but I encourage my patients to push on because the side effects usually decrease over time. I increase the dose of Metformin slowly, usually fortnightly and this has been really effective at preventing side effects.

### THE PILL

The pill is not great for women with IR. On the one hand it regulates your periods when they're all over the show and reduces that heavy bleeding. If you use an anti-androgen or fourth generation pill (see the Hormone Primer) they can really help with excess hair growth and acne as well as hair loss from the top of your head.

The problem is that the oestrogen in the pill also desensitises your insulin receptors. Studies in labs show the pill reduces insulin sensitivity by up to 40 per cent. A recent study of the pill, Yasmin showed it increased blood glucose levels by 20 per cent and we know that type II diabetes is 60 per cent more likely in women on the pill than if they've never taken the pill.

This is a HUGE dilemma for women with PCOS who have an irregular cycle and want all those anti-androgen effects that come from a fourth generation or anti androgen pill but are desperate to lose weight. I usually look at the symptoms and ask my patient what is their greatest concern. If they say weight loss is their first priority we leave off the pill. If the acne and hairiness is their first priority, we start an anti-androgen pill but not until they have had an OGTT and we repeat it six months later. We still start all the other medications (especially Metformin) as well. If six months later the OGTT is worse despite the Metformin and the weight loss is too slow, we stop the pill.

## Extra tips on handling your hormones

### GETTING ORGANISED

You also have to accept that if you just keep eating whatever is on the table you WILL overeat. So you simply MUST lay out your food before you start eating and finish once you hit that limit.

If you've watched *The Biggest Loser* and seen these absolutely enormous people halve their weight in what seems like a single episode, you'd think that anyone can do that in a single day. What you forget is that these people are making a 24 hour job of their weight loss. They're spending eight hours a day with a personal trainer and then working out on their own. They're eating close to zero calories. And they're not broken by screaming kids, the grind of a merciless work life or being stuck in a peak hour gridlock every day.

Sugar cravings, especially in the afternoons, are a real feature of insulin resistance and PCOS. If you don't expect them, if you don't come prepared with an alternative, you will find yourself flagging and unable to concentrate come the afternoon and will feel drawn like a moth to a flame to the kids' treat cupboard at home or the biscuit barrel at work.

Instead, make sure you are prepared. Snacks should always be protein plus carbohydrate to avoid a sugar spike and control your sugar release. Prepare a foil-wrapped hard-boiled egg, a little packet of six unsalted nuts and a piece of fruit or a tub of low-fat (and no added sugar) yoghurt.

### Fix your vitamin D levels

Interestingly, statistically more than 50 per cent of overweight women and 75 per cent of women with PCOS are vitamin D deficient. That is going to be a huge issue in terms of losing weight. For a start, low vitamin D levels can cause muscle weakness, which means your ability to exercise is much lower, so is your ability to lose weight. That is going to aggravate insulin resistance. Vitamin D is absorbed through the skin, but you can take it as a supplement and it does work incredibly well.

If you don't know whether or not you have vitamin D deficiency, see your GP. It is a simple blood test and your GP can advise you whether or not you need a supplement. Just in case you're thinking of bypassing the GP's waiting room and helping yourself to an over-the-counter supplement without knowing your level, I would seriously advise against it. Overdoses of vitamin D do occur and have been linked to heart rhythm problems.

### Stop smoking

Smoking is a no brainer if you have PCOS. Smokers have a higher risk of vascular disease, osteoporosis and mood issues. You're already in the firing line for those problems anyway so anyone with PCOS who still smokes needs their head read. Quit NOW!!

PCOS therapy may take up to six months to get on top of an irregular cycle and hair growth problems (you can consider anything less a bonus). The good news is that mood symptoms often improve within six weeks.

## MANAGE YOUR STRESS

We know that if you are stressed off your head, you may well have relatively elevated levels of cortisol. We also know that cortisol in itself can exacerbate insulin resistance, so being stressed can definitely make it harder to lose weight. Try meditation, talking to a counsellor, exercise and binning those vices, especially alcohol.

## DITCH YOUR ALCOHOL

I have to be honest with you and tell you that there really isn't a link between drinking and your hormones. Except that indirectly there is. Women with IR and PCOS are often really down on themselves, have mood swings and are exhausted. With that combination, it's easy to see how a little tipple at night can turn into a big problem. When you're down and exhausted, it can be hard to stop at a single glass of wine and anecdotally, lots of experts who deal with PCOS and insulin resistance tell me that drinking too much can be a habitual problem for women with these hormonal issues. It is better not to open the bottle so you can remove temptation. We need you sleeping well to augment your hormonal weight loss (see below) and wine can knock off your sleep (See Are My Hormones Making Me Tired?). Plus wine (and other types of alcohol as well) have loads of calories which won't help you with your weight loss.

# Is hormonal sleep deprivation making me fat?

Have you ever noticed that on days after a shocking night's sleep, come 3 pm you could mow down an entire chocolate mousse cake and have room for another? Crave sugar? Crave fat? Become obsessed with food? You might not have been conscious of the connection but think about it; there is a very strong connection between lack of sleep and hunger. That's not only after being a poor sleeper for weeks or even years. It's also after having a single rotten night.

Studies have found a very strong relationship between a chronic lack of sleep and being overweight. People who don't get enough sleep have lower levels of leptin and higher levels of ghrelin (which we covered at the beginning of the chapter.) Which probably explains why sleep deprived people feel hungrier and often crave the very worst foods.

And even our old enemy insulin plays a role with sleep deprivation making insulin sensitivity 16 per cent lower. So being sleep deprived whether short term or long term is going to wreak havoc with your dress size. The way, by the way to manipulate these hormones, apart from getting enough sleep is to… you guessed it… have a healthy diet! A low-fat, low-calorie diet is linked to lower ghrelin and higher leptin levels in the blood.

I'm going to direct you for further information to Are my Hormones Making me Tired? for tips on managing your sleep.

# Is my thyroid making me fat?

If you remember back to our Hormone Primer, the thyroid gland sits at the base of your throat and controls every aspect of your metabolism. It stimulates the break down of fat and carbohydrates from their storage sites, gets them released into the blood stream and encourages your cells to use them. It boosts your heart rate and, as a side effect of so much metabolic activity, it gives off heat. Being that metabolically active, it's no wonder that an underperforming thyroid is linked to weight problems. Of everyone who has a thyroid problem, 80 per cent have an underactive thyroid.

Thyroid problems run in families, so if a member of your family runs into trouble with their thyroid, be on guard for your turn. Your risk also increases with age. Plus we know thyroid problems are around eight times more common in women than men. Having another autoimmune disorder such as diabetes or rheumatoid arthritis can worsen your odds.

We know for sure that an untreated underactive thyroid causes weight gain. But it it's not just the women with low thyroid hormone levels that have an issue. In 2008, a study examining thyroid and weight was done. The researchers found that even a thyroid functioning on the lower end of the normal range is associated with weight gain. For that reason, some clinicians, particularly in the USA do give thyroid hormone supplements to women who have high-normal TSH levels

# Is my menopause making me fat?

Absolutely. I have never met a woman who has sailed through menopause without gaining an extra pound. At least without try-ing damned hard to stay slim. We know from animal studies that oestrogen helps to regulate body weight. If you lower a lab an-imal's oestrogen levels, they not only tend to eat more and be less physically active, but they appear to also have a lower met-abolic rate. Plus we know that oestrogens as part of hormone replacement therapy increase your resting metabolic rate. We think that's at least part of why women gain weight when oestro-gen levels decline after menopause.

It's actually the peri-menopausal years that see women go through a period of relative weight gain. Less oestrogen and more androgens mean that your weight goes straight to your middle (the old spare tyre phenomenon!) instead of your hips and thighs.

Plus we know that after the menopause, with the fall in oestro-gen and the decline in metabolic hormones like the thyroid hor-mone, you probably need to eat about 200 fewer calories a day during your 50s and 60s than you did during your 30s and 40s in order to maintain your current weight.

But before we lay the entire weight gain guilt trip at the feet of your change-of-life hormones, there are other issues at play. Re-search has shown that menopausal women tend to exercise less than other women, which can lead to weight gain.

The other thing that does happen as well is what we call dy-napaenia – or a loss of muscle strength which happens natural-ly as you age. It's not simply that the muscles shrink in volume. Of course they do, but they also change their structure so that they're just less efficient at doing what muscles do.

If you don't do anything to replace the lean muscle you lose, your body composition will shift to more fat and less muscle – which slows down the rate at which you burn calories. If you con-tinue to eat as you always have, you're likely to gain weight.

# How to handle your hormones

When a woman going through menopause comes to me to discuss weight gain, I never assume it's the menopause alone. We know that both an underactive thyroid gland and type II diabetes with its accompanying insulin resistance can all cause weight gain and they're both worth testing for at this stage of life. But assuming they're both OK:

### Exercise of course
Look, this is a bit of a no brainer. But at this time of your life, you can't be hanging up the walking shoes. They're more important than ever. I know you're bleeding heavily, never know when the next period is due, your mood swings are making you cranky and your flashes are stopping you from wanting to do anything that will make you hotter! But if you give up exercising, you will definitely gain more weight. It is that simple.

### Eat less
We know you need to eat fewer calories to maintain your weight. It has to be done. Reduce your portion sizes, fill up on raw veggies, vegetable soup and water, tea and coffee so you don't overeat at meal times.

### Boost your muscle power
A Canadian study of women who had been through the menopause found that the biggest predictor of low muscle strength was lower protein in the diet. That was far more significant than being older, more overweight, or how far down the menopause track you were. So trying to eat more protein in your diet will help boost muscle power to enable you to burn more energy from your workout.

### Hormone replacement Therapy (HRT)
OK this is a BIG can of worms I have just opened here. I have dealt in detail with the ins and outs of HRT in the chapter Are My Hormones Making Me Tired? Nobody advocates using HRT to control your weight. But if you have other symptoms of menopause, and you need to go onto HRT for another reason, weight control might be a side benefit.

# Is the pill making me fat?

It's one of the most common questions I get asked by younger women who start the pill for contraception. They're naturally worried about weight gain because the legend of the pill making you stack on the extra kilos is so grounded in folklore.

So there are two answers I can give you. Well three if you ask the pseudoscientific natural hormone alternative salespeople they'll tell you pumping any hormones into your body isn't natural and causes chemical reactions that lead to a variety of non-specific symptoms including weight gain. Being a scientist first and foremost I'm just going to declare that's wrong and move on.

So back to the two answers, let me give you the sort of answer you will get from most doctors; they will tell you that the pill weight gain link is simply not true. And indeed the pill hasn't been shown in studies to cause any significant amount of weight gain. Certainly nothing above the two kilo level, and most experts believe that the weight gain is a matter of lifestyle not hormones. When you think about it, lots of girls start the pill when they start college or university, right at the time of that famous 'freshman five' phenomenon where kids stack on an average of five pounds in their first year, especially if they've moved away from home and mum's cooking to campus food and masses and masses of alcohol. So, they would tell you, blame the lifestyle morass that plagues the lazy-ass teenagers who quit netball in the last years of high school or their early 20s rather than the pill. I think those stats are true for many cases of weight gain registered while taking the pill.

But here is my second of the two answers: without a doubt there are some girls who do put on weight from the pill. The culprit is a reaction between your baseline hormones and the hormones in the pill IF you have polycystic ovaries and insulin resistance (see above).

For a start, when you start talking to girls with these hormone imbalances, they often report having ballooned up after starting the pill. But secondly we have scientific proof; we know that oestrogen makes the insulin receptors less efficient. Studies have shown that standard oral contraceptive pills reduce insulin sensitivity by a massive 30 to 40 per cent. For ages we have known that it's the skyrocketing oestrogen levels in pregnancy that often bring on diabetes of pregnancy (gestational diabetes). Now admittedly your oestrogen levels on the pill are MUCH lower than they are with pregnancy but they're still quite a bit higher than they are at baseline off the pill. So in girls with PCOS and insulin resistance, being on the pill will raise insulin levels and as a result, it can make them hungrier and shut down fat burning, meaning that the most well intentioned would-be dieter is facing a soul destroying uphill battle to shift even 200 grams.

Now before you throw your pill in the bin, you should have a look at the complexity of the situation. The pill is very handy for women with PCOS. It is often the only way they can have anything resembling normal periods and off the pill, periods will often go back to being incredibly painful and all over the show, which is a serious pain in the neck. Plus if you are using an anti-androgen pill for body hair and acne control, and it's working, it seems a shame to go off it.

For women in this situation, I usually treat the underlying insulin resistance and polycystic ovarian syndrome and ask my patient which of the issues of her PCOS/IR are worrying her the most. If it is the weight gain, we have a go off the pill. If it's the cycle control or the zits or hairiness, we can stay on the pill but do two OGTTs six months apart. If they're getting worse or you have weight gain, we'll have to consider ditching the pill and hoping that aggressive insulin lowering does enough to regulate the cycle and the excess androgen.

Dr Ginni's five weight loss rules for any cause of hormonal (or even non hormonal) weight gain:

### Rule of France

One of my favourite rules. This works! Have you ever been to France? If you're lucky enough to have strolled down a beautiful tree-lined street in gay Paris, or pretty much anywhere else in France for that matter, you will probably be grateful for all the tourists because the locals will make you feel like an elephant. Me included. I have always been fascinated by the fact that the average patisserie (and there are four on every intersection!) empties out by lunchtime and yet French people look like catwalk models. And don't look for joggers. They're pretty thin on the ground! I thought maybe it was just the genes but after a while I worked out something; the French LOVE their food. It is a celebration. You wouldn't catch a French lady standing at the sink scoffing one of the kids' half eaten muffins! Ew! No, if it is worth eating, it is worth putting it on a plate and SITTING at the table. From now on, eat like a Parisienne! No more grabbing a biccie from the biscuit barrel at work while you boil the kettle, no more grabbing some crackers and eating them standing up while you cook dinner! No more standing at the sink eating the kids' cold leftovers. No, from now on, eating is a French celebration. Set the table, put it on a plate and eat it slowly, sitting down and savouring every mouthful.

## Rule of USA

I like the salad first concept that Americans use. Americans often start their meals with a salad. I might not LOVE the type of salad they eat... too much sugar, candied nuts and creamy dressings... but the concept of filling up on salad and veggies before the meat or fish is great. When I ask most of my patients what they had for dinner last night the answer is chicken or roast lamb. The veggies, such as they are, are very much a side line. But we know that it's the meat or fish that should be the added extras to the vegetables. One easy way to do that is to make an entrée of salad like the Americans and once everyone has had a plateful, to move on to the rest of the meal. In winter substitute a warming vegetable soup for a salad.

## Fluid restrictions

There is no reason for anyone watching their weight to drink any drink other than water, tea, coffee or the occasional alcoholic drink. I know that is seriously hard line but I want you to think about the number of calories you consume when you have a drink like a juice. There are about four oranges in the average glass of orange juice. Try eating four oranges and you will struggle, but you can drink them down in five seconds flat which delivers you another entire meal worth of kilojoules, only it doesn't fill you up. If you take a 375 ml bottle of apple juice, it contains seven teaspoons of sugar – eight in a pineapple juice. That's not much better than a soft drink! They are all unnecessary calories that we can do without. People get surprised at my anti-juice stand but there is nothing in a juice that you need. Substitute one glass for a couple of whole pieces, grab yourself the same vitamins but add in the fibre and extra anti-oxidants from the skin that gets omitted in the juicing process and you are going to be far better off. As for soft drinks, they just pack on calories for zero nutritional benefits whatsoever. Soft drinks are linked to obesity, strokes and diabetes. Lots of my patients drop tons of weight just by cutting out soft drinks. Diet drinks are in reserve if you can't stand water. That's because they prime your brain to crave sweet foods so it can make all the other strategies harder.

### Drinking games

Water that is. Women need 2.1 litres of fluid per day ON TOP of your food to stay well hydrated and men need 2.6 litres a day. You only need to be as little as two per cent dehydrated to feel horrible. You are physically and mentally off your game immediately and long term you're also at risk of kidney stones, some cancers and heart problems. If you do nothing to make yourself feel less sluggish than drink an extra couple of glasses of water or cups of tea or coffee a day, it will be a great start. If you hate water, try fizzy water or one of these tips; I love sprigs of fresh mint, or a couple slices of fresh lemon, lime or ginger root or a smashed cardamom pod in my water.

### Not in my back yard. Or home

There is one unbreakable rule for you, your husband and kids; no naughty food in the house. You know why: if it's there, you get hit with a sugar craving whether from sleep deprivation or insulin resistance or just because it's that time of the month and you need the willpower of a saint to keep your hands off that sugary treat. If you're entertaining? Party presents! Send all the cakes and cookies home with your guests. Whatever gets rejected gets binned. And if someone brings you chocolates, then surely there's a teacher at school or a work colleague who you can honour with a regifting of sorts: 'I was given these but I really want you to have them'. By the way, if in doubt bring them to your local GP's surgery where I promise you some of the front desk girls will do justice to the chocolates!! If you know an area where there are lots of homeless people, they will definitely appreciate a box of biccies or chocolates and that is a win-win all round.

# Are My Hormones Making Me Moody?

This is often the crux of the problems patients bring to me. When they tell me they feel 'hormonal', they're often saying they feel moody.

"I get hormonal before my periods."

"My teenager is so hormonal."

"I don't know what's wrong with me; I'm so hormonal all the time."

News flash: your brain controls your moods. But by now you know just how many hormone receptors there are in your brain, so let's look at how your hormones control your mood.

## Hormones and the brain

It will not surprise most women to learn that indeed there is a huge neurobiological link between our hormones and our behaviour. Anyone who experiences the dreaded PMS, AKA premenstrual syndrome, or on the flip side your periods get out of whack and become irregular when you're up to your eyeballs in stress can blame the effect of your hormones on the temporal lobes in your brain. These lobes are located on either side of the brain.

Specifically, it is in the inner or medial portions of the temporal lobe where our emotions and our hormones come together and wreak havoc. That is because the medial parts of our temporal lobes house the hippocampus and the amygdala. These weird-sounding names are actually two important parts of the limbic system, a group of interconnected parts of the brain areas that basically sort through our emotions and allocate the right emotion to certain problems or situations. Your hippocampus sorts out your short term memory while the amygdala is basically where emotional relevance is mapped onto our memories. For example, if you get bitten by a dog, you might experience fear next time you see a dog. That is because your amygdala and hippocampus have colluded to keep you safe and protect you from getting too close to dangerous dogs.

Would it surprise you to find out that the limbic system is also the part of our brains with MOST of the oestrogen and progesterone receptors making them most sensitive to hormonal swings? Aha! The limbic system is also connected to two other vital parts of the brain (featured in the hormone primer); the hypothalamus and pituitary gland, which, as you remember, produce the vital girly hormones. At times of stress, the amygdala and hippocampus can work together to shut down the sex hormones produced by the pituitary and hypothalamus, making your periods go haywire and stopping ovulation or at least make ovulation sporadic. This is obviously your body's way of stopping you from getting pregnant at such a tumultuous time and things often return to normal when the stress settles down and the hippocampus and amygdala work out all is back to normal again.

To look at the relationship between your hormones and your brain more thoroughly, I am going to go through the specific actions of oestrogen and progesterone on your brain. I know we did this very briefly in the Hormone Primer, but here I'll go into a little more detail about how your girly hormones affect your brain and mood.

## Oestrogen – the feel-good hormone

Oestrogen activates the cells in the brain by activating the oestrogen receptors that are, as you now well know, on every cell to a greater or lesser degree. When it comes to brain cells, oestrogen increases the levels of the feel-good brain chemical, serotonin, and at the same time increase the number of serotonin receptors in the brain, meaning not only will you have more feel-good chemicals, but they will work more effectively as well.

Oestrogen also decreases monoamine oxidase (MAO) activity in the brain. MAO is a real downer in your brain. That's because it breaks down your brain's feel good serotonin and noradrenaline. More MAO = misery. So as more oestrogen means less MAO and therefore more of the feel-good serotonin and noradrenaline, it has even more of a feel-good effect.

As well as the serotonin effect, when oestrogen activates the oestrogen receptor, the cells basically speed up. The cell's metabolism accelerates, making it use more sugar and oxygen, its main fuels. Oestrogen also increases blood flow to the brain, ensuring sugar and oxygen are delivered faster. That's why scientists view oestrogen as an 'upper', giving you more energy and elevating your mood.

In case you want to overdose on the stuff, there is an issue. You can get too much of a good thing and too much oestrogen not counterbalanced by progesterone can make you feel very anxious. In extreme situations it can even induce seizures.

## Progesterone – the chill-out hormone

Calming the situation is oestrogen's natural partner, progesterone. Studies have shown that giving either women or men an injection of progesterone makes them feel sleepy and slows down the heart rate. Other studies have shown that women who take cocaine get less of an upper effect in the second half of their cycle when progesterone levels are higher. And giving women progesterone tablets also inhibits the high from cocaine and other drugs.

We're slowly gaining an understanding of HOW progesterone works as a sedative. It all starts with a neurotransmitter called GABA, which effectively works as a tranquiliser. Activating GABA receptors, by the way is how most sedative medicines work. Anyway, progesterone breaks down into allopregnanolone, which, like a sedative medicine basically intensifies the sedative effects of GABA. Immediately after you've given birth, and immediately before a period, progesterone levels pretty much fall off a cliff. As a result you get a huge drop in your blood levels of allopregnanolone. This in turn stops turbo charging GABA to do its thing. Lots of doctors believe that THIS progesterone withdrawal is behind the worst symptoms of premenstrual syndrome or PMS as well as postnatal insomnia and mood. The effect is not dissimilar to withdrawing from a sleeping pill.

## Hormonal imbalance

As you already know by now from reading the Hormone Primer, there are key times in women's lives when hormone imbalances eventuate, in women predisposed to them. And by the way, that is the key – being predisposed to them. Not everybody's brains go troppo when there's a hormone imbalance. But if you are genetically wired with lots of hypersensitive oestrogen receptors in your brain, this might be a problem for you.

The first is around the start of puberty when you first get your periods. Your ovaries are capable of making oestrogen many months before you're capable of ovulating and balancing out your oestrogen with the calming effects of progesterone from the corpus luteum. We know those first few periods that are heavy, painful and irregular when you're a young teenager are probably anovulatory periods – oestrogen but no progesterone. If you know any young girls, on the verge of puberty, you will probably have witnessed first hand the stress and anxiety effect of what we call 'unopposed oestrogen'.

The next time is if and when you go on the pill. The oestrogens in the ill directly act on the brain, but they all contain synthetic progestogens (progestins), which do not have brain activity. No ill contains natural progesterone, which of course has powerful brain activity, and can offset that of the oestrogen. From the brain's point of view, being on the pill is like being in a state of hormone imbalance with 'unopposed oestrogen' in play.

Then it can happen if you get polycystic ovarian syndrome and insulin resistance. Failure to ovulate can lead to a hormonal imbalance with a lack of calming progesterone, which is exacerbated when a female puts on weight (which most but not all) women with PCOS do. That is because the fat cells will convert lots of testosterone to even more oestrogen because of the enzyme aromatase. Plus, because women with PCOS tend to have so much testosterone, there is lots of testosterone available to be converted to oestrogen. It gives you a major hormone imbalance.

The last time is when a woman is at the end of her fertile life, the peri-menopause AKA hormone hell. Again, her ovaries are able to make oestrogen but without ovulating or if the ovulation produces a substandard corpus luteum, there will be little to no counterbalancing progesterone to calm her mood. And again, too much aromatase, care of too much body fat, will make the problem worse. Mood swings are such a huge part of the peri-menopause and 'unopposed oestrogen' certainly plays a role.

### CORTISOL

We met cortisol back in the Hormone Primer, but it has to be visited again. It is a steroid hormone released in response to stress by the adrenal glands in response to stimulation by the ACTH from your hypothalamus in your brain. Its effects include breakdown and degeneration of nerves in the brain, especially the areas responsible for mood, memory and thinking. It also suppresses your ability to sleep.

Cortisol is also known as the age-acceleration hormone. It breaks down collagen and elastin (the connective tissues in your skin), causing wrinkles as well as aches and pains in your muscles, joints and bones. It also shuts down your thyroid, your sex hormones and the sensitivity of your insulin receptors. It also causes cell death of the cells in your brain. The death of certain cells in your brain may also be responsible for your mood swings.

In every study of stress reduction strategies, it is cortisol levels that are used to monitor how well you respond or otherwise.

### ALLOPREGNANOLONE

This hormone is relatively new in terms of discovery and understanding. We know it actively binds our GABA receptors in the brain, activating them and serving as a tranquiliser. If you remember back to the Hormone Primer, there are basically two sources; one is as a breakdown product from progesterone, which sees it rise along with progesterone in the second half of the cycle. The second is from the adrenal glands in response to stress to calm us down when our bodies are preparing for a fight or flight response.

Returned servicemen with PTSD have low levels of pregnenolone. Interestingly, it is thought that teenagers' brains can have this ironic response to allopregnanolone where it makes them MORE anxious rather than less. Check this theory out later when we talk about teenage mood swings.

If these hormone swings affect the brain so much, how come we're not ALL raving loonies before our cycle? (And if you're a man and IF you're saying YES you all are...just shut up. We're not interested!!) Apart from the way your own individual genes regulate the number, position and sensitivity of the various hormone receptors, there is another theory: the hormones fluxes affect some of us more than others based on our genes and based on our underlying personalities.

# Are hormones making my teenager moody?

Do you have a teenager at home? I have lots. Sam, my son, is now 20, meaning we have only three teens for the time being until Jodi and Tara get older. But believe me, with six kids in the house, we know all about teenage moods.

Let's go through what's going on in your teenager's brain:
First of all, allopregnanolone which we met in the Hormone Primer does something seriously whacky in teenagers. In adults and young children it activates the GABA receptor and is a little tranquiliser. But for some reason, in teens it has this opposite effect. The reason for this is that there are a few types of allopregnanolone receptors in the brain and only one type (which is almost absent in kids and adults) blocks GABA and increases anxiety – while the rest do the opposite. That receptor makes a brief appearance at puberty so your teen is not so much tranquilised as angst-ridden by their calm-down hormones! Poor things!

In girls we have our old friend, the oestrogen-progesterone imbalance. Until her cycle becomes regular and she starts ovulating, she will have unopposed oestrogen making her stressed.

The other reasons for the mood swings are more likely to be non hormonal. Bad diet, lack of sleep and growth of different parts of the brain at different times are also factors.

## How to handle your teenager's hormones

### MORE SLEEP

Teenagers need eight and a quarter to nine and a half hours sleep per night. Is your teenager getting that? In my practice, few teens come close. With their crazy schedules and mountains of homework, they're only left with the wee hours to Facebook, Instagram, Tumblr, Tweet and text each other.

Take a look at your teen's schedule and cleave off unnecessary activities. And get a techno ban happening from 9 pm each night to help them get more time to sleep. That means giving mum the iPhone, smartphone, iPad, laptop and gaming controls at 9 pm on condition of strict privacy. You must swear not to fish through their messages no matter how tempting. They can have them all returned each morning when they wake up.

### MORE EXERCISE

With all the thumb action they're getting on their phones and all the bum action they're getting when using their laptops, it's hard to believe they need any more workout time right? Teens need to burn off energy and their mood swings are reduced by exercise. Doesn't need to be an expensive ballet class with you as chauffeur. Give them the dog to run after school for a half hour round trip!

### DETOX

Hey I'm not advocating stupid, non scientific, expensive, supplement riddled detoxes. I'm all for more water, fruit, veggies, lean meat, dairy and fish and less processed rubbish. Teens sometimes have the weirdest diets. It's like they want to follow Gwyneth Paltrow but add in a kilo of Mars Bars and Twisties as supplements. If you can help them make the link between their shocking diet and their moods, (plus their skin and weight), they might be more open to changing their diet. But you have to lead from the front. Don't have rubbish in the house, don't pack it in their lunch boxes and don't eat it yourself!

TEEN EMPOWERMENT

This is a fundamental parenting style issue, but I like to take the reins off and empower my kids to make good decisions. This is a time where teens like to be the masters of their own destiny. They will fail sometimes. But if you assume that they're so stupid and have such poor judgement that you can't let them out of your sight lest they wreck their futures with their appalling behaviour, you're sending some pretty negative messages to them and to their friends. Give as much rope as is safe and allow them to prove themselves as responsible nearly-adults. Gradually give them more freedom and responsibility with lots of encouragement and positive feedback. I promise you will get a better response from them than the frustration that comes from being kept in a cage.

MANAGING THEIR ALCOHOL

We have faced this demon in our home a lot. In some western countries, a culture has developed among teens where getting smashed on alcohol is a pre-requisite to having a good night. We are not talking a couple of beers. We're talking ten plus shots of vodka. I'm going to give you my advice as a parent and a doctor. There is NOTHING ok about this. Heavy drinking kills off their brain cells at a time they need to study, it damages their internal organs and places them at risk of violent clashes, getting run over and of sexual violence. Plus in the age of Instagram where their public humiliation is even more public, the humiliation can last for years.

But at the same time, a culture of honesty within families, while always important, is VITAL at this time. Once trust has broken down, the ramifications for the rest of your relationship can be devastating. So if you say that getting drunk is so bad that if you find out they've been drunk, they'll be grounded for a year, you will almost force them to lie to you and sneak behind your back and the damage will be worse.

What to do? There is no quick fix here. One small step at a time. Focus on your relationship with your children from day one. If you are someone to whom they look up, whose advice they value, and who they do not want to disappoint, then there's a good chance of having great communication. They will trust that you're not some clueless clot hell bent on destroying their fun. But rather see you as a smart, caring, switched on role model whose advice is worth taking.

Apart from giving them the same messages about safe drinking, you need to ensure they're safe. That they can call you if in trouble. That they go everywhere with a friend and look out for each other. That they sms you to let you know they're safe and where they are. That they've had something to eat before they go out. Discuss using social media wisely. Never buy alcohol for your kids as that's buying in to their heavy drinking. Never host drinking for under aged teenagers as their friends' parents might rightly be pretty upset about that. Apart from that, hope your kids are sensible and well-brought up enough to drink sensibly and avoid trouble.

### Get help

If your teenager is withdrawing from friends, moving crowds to a completely inappropriate group, being hostile or locking themselves in their room, don't assume it's 'just hormones.' Serious mental health issues in teens are under recognized because they do get labelled as hormonal issues. If in ANY doubt, get him or her to a trained psychologist and ask a professional to check them out.

# Is my PMS making me moody?

Feel like rubbish just before your period? It must be one of the commonest complaints I hear in my practice. Premenstrual syndrome or PMS is a favourite of men who like to call their partners irrational and hormonal in an argument. But it's real and it can be devastating.

About a week ago one of my patients came in to see me and told me as calmly as you please that three days before her last period she had grabbed a carving knife from the kitchen shelf during an argument with her hubby and had every intention of using it on his head!

Statistics suggest that around 90 per cent of us women report experiencing at least one unpleasant symptom before a period. When these symptoms (whatever they are) come on like clockwork before your period and at levels enough to interfere with your life, you have premenstrual syndrome (PMS). PMS is super common and depending on how you define it, anywhere from ten to 40 per cent of women are sufferers. There are some women whose symptoms (see below) are severe enough to interfere with their ability to live their life. The symptoms typically start after ovulation, so anywhere between one and two weeks before your period starts. And most importantly, they disappear altogether when your period finishes. The other important feature of PMS is its predictability. Occasional symptoms don't cut it for a diagnosis of PMS.

The sorts of symptoms we are taking about include both the physical and the emotional variety.

Most women know the physical symptoms: bloating, swelling especially of the breasts – think an extra cup size on your bra! Swelling in the arms or legs and breast tenderness. But other symptoms include muscle aches, attack of the killer pimples, headaches, feeling moody, being 'emotional' (bursting into tears at the drop of a hat) as well as more extreme symptoms like depression, irritability, anxiety and even social withdrawal. But it can include food cravings, fatigue, abdominal pains, gas, etc. In fact over 150 symptoms have been linked with PMS. The most severe form of emotional PMS is premenstrual dysphoric disorder (PMDD). Basically what distinguishes PMDD is the severity of emotional symptoms, such as marked depression and anxiety. But it's all part of the same problem.

Here's something interesting; if you're not ovulating, you won't get PMS. So if being fertile and ovulating matters to you, at least your PMS is telling you that indeed your little lady friends are functioning like little troopers and making you some lovely eggs each month!

# What causes PMS?

Will it surprise you to hear we still don't fully understand it but some clear risk factors have been identified:
* Emotional stress
* Bad eating habits
* Experiencing nasty side effects on the pill

* Drinking too much (alcohol)
* Having excess salt in the diet
* Having a high sugar diet
* A high intake of caffeine
* Being a smoker
* Having a history of depression
* Having experienced pre-eclampsia or eclampsia during your pregnancy
* Having a family history of PMS or depression
* Being aged over 30

As time has gone on and more studies have been done, more and more of the symptoms of PMS are being blamed on a hormone – progesterone. If you remember back to our Hormone Primer, it's the second half of the cycle that sees your progesterone levels surge courtesy of the corpus luteum. Progesterone definitely relaxes the smooth muscles in the walls of the veins, which makes them more prone to leaking out fluid and so is most likely responsible for the swelling in the tummy, hands and feet as well as breast tenderness. You know already that progesterone decreases the brain's output of serotonin and changes the way serotonin acts in the brain. We know from separate research that lower levels of serotonin activity in the brain causes flat mood, irritability, anger, aggression, poor impulse control, and cravings for carbohydrates.

But we all get hormonal fluxes around our cycle. So why do only some women get PMS? The current theory dominating this field is that some of us are genetically primed to have more extreme reactions to these hormonal changes. Hence the fact that PMS often runs in families.

There are no tests for PMS, which can be frustrating for some women. But what I find is the most effective way to be sure that your problem is PMS is to keep a two-month symptom diary to track the symptoms and their severity, then tick them off against the time of the cycle.

# How to handle your PMS hormones

### EXERCISE

The jury is now in. As long as your PMS is not interfering with your daily life, exercise is the best place to start treating PMS. Exercise has been shown in multiple studies to be highly effective in reducing the symptoms of PMS pretty much across the board, it is good for you in so many other ways in addition to relieving the symptoms of PMS and is side effect free! What the jury is still out on is how much and what type. Experts suggest 30 minutes five days a week of an exercise YOU enjoy. Walking, swimming, jogging, Zumba, pilates, boot camp – it's your call. Just get off the couch and move.

### CHASTE BERRY (*VITEX AGNUS-CASTUS*)

Chaste berry is the berry of the chaste tree and has a long history of use for all sorts of female hormonal problems. In almost all studies there's no evidence to support its use, except for PMS. For this condition there evidence from small but well conducted randomised controlled studies, especially around reducing breast swelling and tenderness, swelling, mood swings, anger and headache. The required dose is around 4 mg a day. There are very few side effects, (no more than with a placebo) and it doesn't interact with other medicines (except for some used in Parkinson's disease, which women with PMS don't tend to have). It is definitely worth a shot.

### GO ON THE PILL (AHEM MAYBE)

The theory behind taking an oral contraceptive is to get rid of cycle-related fluctuations in oestrogen and progesterone. You can skip 'periods' on the pill by skipping the sugar pills and moving straight onto the next pack without having a bleed. It's completely safe and can minimise the fluctuations further. Don't forget you can have some breakthrough spotting after a few months so some women prefer to skip one or two periods at a time and just endure the PMS on the third cycle. However, bottom line it only works for a minority of women. Unfortunately studies show that only about a quarter of women who start the pill get any symptom relief at all. But half report no improvement, and the remainder of women actually find the pill makes their symptoms worse.

155

### Change your pill

In the Hormone Primer, I talked about the different progestogens used in different pill formulations. Some newer, fourth generation pills use drospirenone – specifically the pills Yasmin and Yaz. Drospirenone is a close relative of an interesting medication called spironolactone (see below). Spironolactone is not only a diuretic, which helps shed water that contributes to bloating and breast tenderness, but it also has some anti-androgen properties, so it is marketed for women who suffer from acne. But more importantly, Yaz has been shown specifically to be effective for the treatment of the mood swings of PMS. If you are taking anti-inflammatory tablets, diuretics, blood-pressure pills, or potassium supplements chat to your GP about having your blood potassium levels checked early on in your treatment.

### Get plenty of sleep

Everything is worse when you're on your nose with exhaustion. I can't tell you how many of my patients find that they get teary if their kids go through a bad spell of sickness (or naughtiness!) and are up through the night for weeks on end. It's not depression. It's frank exhaustion. But with the exhaustion, everything they might have usually shrugged off becomes an insurmountable mountain. Aim for eight hours for as many nights as you can and just see whether that makes a difference. It won't cure your PMS but it might tip it back from unmanageable to doable.

### See a counsellor

We know that women who are stressed experience much worse PMS than women with not a whole lot of worry in their life. I know EVERYONE is stressed and lots of us are handling our relationships, work, anxiety-provoking parents and children but sometimes we don't register the IMPACT it's having until something as silly as a little PMS makes your work day and family life a chore. You might only be feeling your stress in breast tenderness and wanting to shove a fork in your husband's eye for watching the footy instead of helping you vacuum the lounge but I can promise you, it's running havoc all over your life. From lower immune system functioning to a higher risk of major depression and heart disease, stress isn't simply a trite first-world problem. Take this opportunity to use the PMS as an excuse to make EVERYTHING better.

### CUT BACK ON SALT

We know women who have a high-salt diet retain more fluid AND suffer more PMS. While it is not the cause in all women it is definitely worth cutting back on your salt and seeing if the swelling improves. You would need to try this for at least two months to be sure it's having an effect. Salt isn't just the stuff you add at the table. Basically anything processed from crackers and breakfast cereals to cookies and spreads are packed with salt. Recent studies have shown that the salt content of processed foods has skyrocketed in recent times. We've become immune to the taste of salt but not the physical effects. Cutting it down by ditching processed foods can be hard. As can cutting down the salt in your cooking. Initially everything tastes totally blahhhh. But you get used to it eventually.

### CUT BACK ON SUGAR

I'm a big fan of limiting processed simple sugars anyway. I'm not saying cut them out altogether. I'm not a sadist and I'm not unrealistic. But you don't need to be a rocket scientist to work out that sugar, whether in the form of sports drinks or soft drinks, jelly snakes, cakes, sugary breakfast cereals or ice cream, does your brain no favours. And research showing that people who vacuum up the sweet stuff get more PMS just adds more weight to the instruction to save sugar for a special treat only.

### LIMIT YOUR ALCOHOL

We know women who drink too much get more PMS. In studies women who drank more than ten drinks per week had the highest levels of PMS. I have found in practice that for many of my patients, there is this massive disconnect between how much they drink and what they think of their drinking. Let me explain: if I ask my patients, very few of them think they drink too much. But their version of non-problem drinking and mine is often pretty different. Both men and women should drink no more than two 'standard drinks' each containing 10 grams of alcohol per day. You'll get 10 grams of alcohol from a can of light (lower alcohol) beer or

100 ml of either red or white wine. Try pouring that amount into a measuring beaker and then putting it in your wine glass at home. With 750 ml in the average wine bottle, each bottle should pour seven and a half glasses of wine. If you're only getting four glasses to a bottle, then you're having closer to two standard drinks per glass so your two glasses of wine is like four standard drinks – which is way too much. .

### Quit smoking
Again this is a win-win for your entire body, soul, aroma and wallet. Cigarettes have absolutely no upside. There's not even one healthy cigarette you can have. Women are often surprised to hear that being a smoker can contribute to their PMS. My thought is that while the threat of heart disease and cancer would motivate me a tad more, if beating the bloating mood swings is motivation enough for you to quit cigarettes, I'll take it. Get rid of the cigarettes. Chat to your GP about ways to quit including patches, gums, mists and tablets as well as a plethora of counselling and support tools.

### Bin the liquorice
If you're screwing up your face in disgust at the mere thought of liquorice, you have nothing to worry about. But lovers of the black sweet stuff (like me!) will retain fluid if you have enough of it and that certainly won't help your boobs or bloating.

### Fish oil
A small study of 120 women with PMS found they benefited more with beating their symptoms from a single one gram tablet containing a blend of healthy omega three fats (like the ones in a fish oil capsule) per day than from a placebo. I'm a big fan of fish oil anyway for its anti-inflammatory properties. There are close to no side effects and it won't harm you. The dose would be 2000 mg (or two standard fish oil capsules) per day right through the cycle.

### Avoid diet soft drinks
In a large US study of almost 300,00 adults, the ones who drank four or more cups or cans of diet soft drink per day were 30 per

cent more likely to develop depression than those who drank no soft drinks. We don't know why that's the case or whether there's some nasty ingredient in diet soft drinks that affects the brain. But this study adds weight to the unease most health professionals have about these drinks.

## Specific treatments for specific symptoms within PMS

While there are 150 symptoms associated with PMS, often it's one simple symptom that causes a particular sufferer the most grief. Or alternately, sometimes all the symptoms are so severe that they need to be targeted separately.

### ANTI-DEPRESSANTS FOR PMS – FOR MOOD SWINGS (AND MORE)

They work. There are thousand of clinical trials for popular anti-depressants for PMS and in over 60 per cent of PMS sufferers, there is a huge reduction in moodiness (admittedly there's also over 30 per cent improvement with a placebo). It's the girls with a wide range of physical AND mood issues who see the greatest improvement, rather than the girls with mainly physical symptoms. Plus girls with the most severe symptoms also benefit most. Anti-depressants aren't for everyone but if moodiness from PMS is taking a toll on your life, you should consider giving them a try.

### SPIRONOLACTONE – FOR FLUID RETENTION AND BLOATING

Spironolactone is a diuretic, which means it gets the kidneys to help eliminate excess fluid from the body. It also looks and acts so much like a steroid hormone that it has been found to have some very specific anti-androgen activity, especially working to help reduce hair loss in women. (See Are My Hormones Making Me Look Bad?) Studies of spironolactone for PMS in general have had hopeless results, but it remains the drug of choice to combat bloating and other features of fluid retention – because anecdotally they do work, even though the individual experiences aren't backed up by large-scale trials. Each tablet is usually 25 mg and you would take one in the morning when symptoms are bad or for seven to ten days prior to your period. There are few side effects but it does shift the chemical balance in your body in favour of potassium. So never take a potassium supplement with it.

### ANTI-INFLAMMATORIES FOR PAIN

These medications like ibuprofen and diclofenac are fantastic for managing the physical symptoms like back pain, period pains and joint aches and pains. If your periods are regular and your symptoms are consistent, you can start taking them the day before the symptoms are due. Different anti-inflammatories have different dosing regimens so follow the directions on the packet carefully and always have them with food as they can irritate the stomach.

# The jury is out

### ACUPUNCTURE

If you're vaguely remembering some studies supporting the use of acupuncture for PMS, you'd be spot on. The problem is that the quality of the studies has been so universally poor, and hampered by bias, that scientists say they can't conclude that acupuncture is any better than a placebo. Acupuncture is not cheap so if money is tight and you're not happy to part with hard-earned cash for a possible placebo, you had better think twice. But if you don't care whether it's a real effect or a placebo and you have the money and get a benefit, good for you. Just ensure that your acupuncturist uses clean, disposable needles and preferably is well qualified.

### VITAMIN B6

This vitamin is involved in the synthesis of some of the feel-good neurotransmitters in the brain, which is why it has been postulated as a good supplement for PMS. Everyone has been excited by the ONE well designed, placebo-controlled study of vitamin B6 supplements at a dose of 100 mg daily for sufferers of PMS which showed great symptom reductions for sufferers of PMS. Unfortunately the other, subsequent studies of B6 for PMS, (and there have been lots) haven't managed to replicate these results, casting a shadow over the true efficacy of these supplements. Plus, what we do know is that in high doses (>600 mg/day), vitamin B6 therapy has been found to damage some of the nerves especially of the feet – causing a nasty condition known as peripheral neuropathy. The bottom line is that if you stick to the dosing on the packaging, B6 supplements are unlikely to hurt you. If you try it and find it works at safe levels, keep going!

### Calcium supplements

Again we're faced with some conflicting data. One small study in 1998 found that PMS symptoms were reduced by 48 per cent in women taking 1,200 milligrams of calcium a day, compared with a 30 per cent reduction in women taking a placebo. But in 2005 a subsequent study found that women who ate more dairy products had less PMS, but the same couldn't be said of women taking calcium supplements. I don't have a problem with anyone wanting to give calcium supplements a go for PMS. A 2012 study did link calcium supplements with heart attacks in older women- but 70 plus ladies don't need PMS assistance!

### Magnesium supplements

Here we are on even thinner ice than with calcium. In a couple of studies, taking magnesium supplements, at a dose of between 200 and 400 mg per day was helpful in relieving PMS symptoms. However, as the studies were of very poor quality indeed, we can't be sure the results seen in those trials were not simply a placebo effect. Having said that, if you want to take magnesium supplements and you feel they work for you, go for it. Just beware that they can give you a mild laxative effect if you take them in higher doses

### Evening primrose oil

The oil from the seeds of the evening primrose (*Oenothera biennis*) is rich in a chemical called gamma-linolenic acid, which is involved in the body's synthesis of the inflammatory chemical, prostaglandin. The theory behind its use is that women with PMS are lacking in gamma-linolenic acid and therefore get abnormalities in their prostaglandins, which the theory says is linked to PMS. But once again the studies of evening primrose oil are inconsistent and inconclusive. The two trials of the highest quality showed that evening primrose oil was no better than a placebo. Evening primrose oil is safe and if you want to give it a try and find it beneficial, that's a reasonable way to go.

### St John's wort

St John's wort, also known as *Hypericum* is a popular supplement for depression and anxiety and a single small study indeed did find that St John's wort can help reduce both the physical and emotional symptoms of PMS. Women on the herbal supplement reported less cramps, irritability, food cravings, and breast tenderness. The dose is 300 mg three times a day with meals. If you use it properly it's very safe and – apart from some minor tummy upset and your skin becoming more sensitive to sunlight (so burning more easily) – there are few nasty side effects. BUT (and this is a big but) you should never take it without checking with your doctor first. It interacts with so many medications including the pill, antidepressants and antihistamines and it should never be taken if you're thinking about becoming pregnant.

# How not to handle your hormones

### Progesterone supplements

This is a case in point about why scientific studies are actually important BEFORE you put yourself on an unproven treatment. Even recently, women were being prescribed progesterone as vaginal or rectal suppositories for PMS. Apart from the eww factor, the treatment was based completely on uncontrolled studies. When proper studies were done, results proved that in fact progesterone is no better than a placebo for PMS. Plus with newer research showing that it is in fact the progesterone that is responsible for most of the physical and emotional symptoms of PMS, giving progesterone supplements would only give you MORE breast tenderness, bloating, leg and finger swelling and mood swings. It's a giant no-no.

### GnRH agonists

Back we go to science nerd world with our Hormone Primer, and you will remember that the hormone GnRH stimulates the pituitary to release FSH and LH which kick start the ovarian cycle. With GnRH agonist injections, the pituitary gets desensitised to the body's real GnRH making it resistant to stimulation by this hormone. As a result the ovary winds down and basically stops functioning. If this sounds awfully similar to menopause, you're right. So while studies have found these shots do reduce the symptoms of PMS by 75 percent, you simply replace them with the side effects of menopause: hot flashes, insomnia and mood swings. These tend to improve significantly over time and many women say they are less severe than the PMS they were taken for. But with a regimen that induces menopause, there is a higher risk of developing both osteoporosis and heart disease long term so they can only be used for six months maximum. And they tend to be kept for the most extreme cases, not for the majority of women.

### WILD YAM

Wild yam root (*Dioscorea villosa*) contains a chemical called diosgenin, which is actually used in the laboratory to make synthetic steroid hormones. It is in a few herbal combos marketed for the treatment of PMS. They work on the rationale that diosgenin will be converted in the body into progesterone, which would relieve premenstrual symptoms. Well firstly, the breakdown of diosgenin into progesterone has been seen in a petrie dish without any evidence it happens in the human body. But I guess more importantly, the whole progesterone caper is old school and we know that's going to do more harm than good. Anyway, wild yam hasn't been studied for PMS and I wouldn't try it.

### DONG QUAI

This is a favourite of TCM (Traditional Chinese Medicine) practitioners. Dong quai (*Angelica polymorpha* var *sinensis*) is a Chinese herb used in a whole range of secret women's business issues, including PMS. That's despite the fact that there are no decent studies of it, especially for PMS. But my reason for black banning it is that dong quai is not safe for use during pregnancy due to a high risk of miscarriage, so doctors advise it should not be taken by sexually active women unless you're on an excellent form of contraception.

### BLACK COHOSH

This herbal treatment has traditionally been used for all sorts of women's health issues, especially menopause. It is often recommended for women for PMS but has NEVER been trialled for PMS.

It is pretty safe overall but reports of liver damage have freaked out many women and their doctors. It has to be said that there are thousands of women who use black cohosh and very few with liver damage from it but you have to be aware of the risks. And for a supplement without a shred of evidence behind it – not even a single dodgy study, it's just not the way to go.

# Is my (peri-) menopause making me moody?

Headed down the fun journey towards the Change of Life? Feeling moody? Hey! That's all part of the fun. Luckily, most women experiencing the joys of the peri-menopause will do so without any major mental health issues. But one in every five women will develop a case of depression at some point during this time. Yep, that's an increase over the normal rate of depression, which is slightly lower at one in six women.

Having read and understood the peri-menopausal hormone hell, it won't surprise you to read that once you do reach the other side of the rainbow, there may not be a pot of gold, but the rate of depression does actually decrease. The enormous Penn Ovarian Aging Study, confirmed that it's the road TO menopause that is linked to depression but that life after established menopause is blessedly less prone to the Black Dog. This was backed up by another huge US study called the Harvard Study of Moods and Cycles, which looked at women aged between 36 and 44 years with no previous depression and followed them for nine years. The researchers confirmed that it's the peri-menopause that is the culprit. Of course, this makes sense in light of the oestrogen progesterone imbalance we discussed in the Hormone Primer. Once you are menopausal, you have less of everything, which is at least a hormone balance if not ideal!

In a recent study of women who were peri-menopausal and in the early stages of menopause, they were found to have very high cortisol levels. The worse their menopausal symptoms, the higher their cortisol levels. You'd think maybe the stress of severe menopausal symptoms would be the culprit, but the researchers have said that rather, these high cortisol levels could be the cause of many of the symptoms, especially around mood and sleep. When you think that cortisol levels in these high ranges age you, inside and out, it's something you would want to be in control of.

# Which hormones are to blame?

If you are in the early stages of menopause you will have an oestrogen progesterone imbalance. Similarly, if you are well through the menopause but have put on a lot of weight and therefore have a lot of active aromatase in your body (remember that aromatase in fat converts androgens to oestrogen), you could be in a state of oestrogen imbalance. Without the calming effects of progesterone, you are more at risk of feeling stressed and anxious and, ultimately, of getting mood swings.

Lack of sleep could also be a part of the problem. In fact we know that insomnia in peri-menopause is a strong predictor of depression and anxiety in the same period.

## How to handle your hormones

### HIT THE SACK BABY

Get your sleep sorted. Amnesty International has described the practice of sleep deprivation as "cruel, inhuman and degrading treatment" and wants it totally banned under the Geneva Convention. Hear! Hear! It always staggers me the number of people who put up with this sort of cruel, inhuman punishment night in night out without getting help. Snapping at everyone? Feel exhausted? Look ten years older than your age? Feel even older? Ploughing through the pantry like a crazed locust? Little car prangs? Hello? As Dr Phil would say; "how's that working out for you?"

Anyone who knows me knows I am a passionate campaigner for better sleep for all. Not just quantity but quality as well. But both need your focus. Head back to Are My Hormones Making Me Tired? For some guaranteed strategies.

### HRT

So many of my girlfriends and patients hear HRT and start shaking their heads before I can get the words out. But here are your facts; oestrogen replacement therapy for postmenopausal women has been shown in multiple trials to yield huge improvements in your sense of well-being as well as a big decline in depression scores. Plus, oestrogen seems to augment the response to antidepressant treatment for postmenopausal women with depression.

### TIBOLONE

We're really familiar now with the HRT alternative, tibolone. It is a medication which, when broken down by the body, produces a chemical that sits on your oestrogen receptors and activates (some but not all of) them so you get many of the benefits of HRT but with less risk of breast cancer and endometrial cancer. Unlike HRT, tibolone decreases your Sex Hormone Binding Globulin or SHBG levels so that you get more active hormones in the blood. It also has androgen effects, not just oestrogen effects and this extra androgen activity is thought to be responsible for some of the other benefits, especially improved libido. See Are My Hormones Destroying My Sex Life?

Studies have shown that tibolone is incredibly effective for managing mood swings during menopause. I guess the one down side is that you have to wait until you have not had a period for a year to go onto tibolone because of the increased risk of irregular vaginal bleeding in women who don't wait out the year. That can mean you won't get benefit when some women need it most. But it is a good option if mood swings are still hanging around after menopause.

### HAVE A CAPPUCCINO OR FOUR

In a large US study, women who drank two to three cups of caffeinated coffee a day were 15 per cent less likely to develop depression over the 10-year study period, compared with women who drank one cup or less per day. Upping that number to four or more cups of coffee a day lowered the risk by 20 per cent. Unfortunately decaf drinkers didn't get the same benefits. This was just another in a long line of studies linking coffee drinking to a better mood. Good news if you're a fan of the cappuccino!

# The jury is out

### BLACK COHOSH

We already met this member of the buttercup family for PMS. If you remember, it contains a number of compounds that in a petrie dish mimic oestrogen. But studies haven't shown that black cohosh has any effect on actual hormone levels for women in peri-menopause or after the menopause. We're not 100 per cent sure whether it has a role to play here at all. There have definitely been some studies that do suggest that black cohosh can help with menopausal symptoms including the mood swings but other studies have suggested it isn't much better than a placebo. The differing results are in part due to the varying study designs and short study durations but there is another issue because different formulations of black cohosh are used in different studies and the way they measured the improvements were different. But if you want to give black cohosh a try and you're feeling like your mood swings are impossible, chat to your GP. There have been some reports of liver damage (see above). Also, while cloud hangs over the effect of black cohosh on breast cancer, you need to ensure you avoid it if you've ever had breast cancer or if you have a family history of breast cancer.

### Dehydroepiandrosterone (DHEA) supplements

Oooh we are in controversial territory here. There have been six studies published analysing the effects of DHEA on mood and well-being in women. Five out of the six trials reported a positive effect of DHEA on mood and wellbeing. But all the studies again were flawed in their implementation making a really good analysis difficult. Plus there are no LONG TERM studies so we just have no idea whether there are negative consequences from taking it for a long time.

But I've spoken to doctors, especially in the USA who have used DHEA supplements for their patients with menopausal mood swings, libido loss and for weight loss and they swear by it. It is being used more and more. It is available on prescription from your doctor but is not covered by the PBS so is a bit expensive.

Because DHEA can be converted into testosterone in the body it can have some unwanted side effects including body and facial hair. It can also make you irritable and anxious. It can also increase your risk of heart disease and raise your blood pressure.

Talk to your GP about it- and never order anything off the net without consulting a health professional first.

# Is the pill giving me mood swings?

Mood swings probably only affect about two per cent of women who go on the pill but if you are one of those two per cent, it can be an absolute nightmare. I can't tell you how many women see me complaining of mood swings on the pill. They are absolutely convinced that the pill is to blame for wanting to drive a forklift into their boyfriend's face. Well we've already established that hormones have a big effect on the brain and the pill is a hormone tablet. It has synthetic oestrogens and progestogens.

Interestingly, unlike the chill-out natural progesterone, the synthetic progestogens in the pill have no brain activity whatsoever. Not the same story for the oestrogens in the pill which do have brain activity. So women on the pill effectively get full on effects of oestrogen without the opposing effects of progesterone. If you get moody on the pill, it is probably for this reason.

Synthetic progestogens were actually developed to get around the problem that natural progesterone breaks down in the body very quickly and is very expensive to produce. Effectively it isn't viable as a medicine. So scientists have modified progesterone or testosterone to get progestins and we're getting better at it all the time. The newer generations are generally more active and you get less interaction with other types of receptors, which are both advantages. Drospirenone, (the fourth generation progesterone in Yaz and Yasmin), for example has been found to boost endorphin levels in both the brain and the blood which might be why they are beneficial for PMS.

So if you think that your pill is to blame for your mood swings, it would be worthwhile trying a different pill. Trying a fourth generation drospirenone containing pill may improve your mood. But sometimes you simply cannot be on the pill because of the effective oestrogen- progesterone imbalance. If this is the case, we would give you a trial off the pill. If this doesn't resolve the problem very quickly, we would have to consider the possibility that you actually have an underlying depressive illness and that the pill wasn't the culprit at all. In this case you do need to consider other options including counselling, exercise, St John's wort, or, if it is more severe depression, an anti-depressant medicine.

# Are my Polycystic Ovarian Syndrome and insulin resistance making me moody?

We already discussed PCOS and insulin resistance pretty comprehensively when we took a look at Are My Hormones Making Me Fat? As you have read, 50 per cent of women with PCOS and insulin resistance have some sort of mood issue as well. A recent meta-analysis of the data around PCOS and anxiety yielded some interesting results. It seems that women with PCOS and IR are five times as likely to experience some anxiety symptoms as women without these issues. They found anxiety affects 20 percent of women with PCOS versus only four percent in women without the disorder and PCOS sufferers have a nearly sevenfold increase in the risk of generalised anxiety disorder. You are also more likely to suffer from social phobia or obsessive compulsive disorder if you have PCOS.

The reason is largely hormonal. As you will remember, with PCOS you don't ovulate as much, getting trapped for weeks to months at a time in a state resembling the first half of the menstrual cycle where there is a predominance of the upper oestrogen without the counterbalancing chill- out of progesterone. In any condition of unbalanced oestrogen dominance, you can get an overload of stress and anxiety, which can ultimately carve a path straight to mood swings and depression. This oestrogen progesterone imbalance is made worse if you are overweight because the high aromatase enzymes from your fat are busily converting testosterone to oestradiol, the most potent of the oestrogens.

Plus, as Dr Mark Beale, who specialises in the management of these conditions pointed out to me, women with PCOS often feel really down about their looks. Whether it's the acne, the hair loss or the weight gain, these girls often dread going out for a big night, knowing they won't look the way they want to.

Studies have shown that if you focus first on correcting the insulin resistance, a better mood is one of the first and most noticeable affects. In most cases if you have both low mood and the PCOS insulin resistance combo, treating the PCOS and IR and correcting those major hormone imbalances will yield much greater benefits than simply taking an antidepressant and focusing on the brain alone.

See your GP. To my great sadness, lots of GPs don't understand either PCOS or IR. I can't believe the number of women I see who have been hammered by their hormones for years and have been fobbed off and told there's nothing that can be done for their mood swings other than taking anti-depressant medications. Hey, forget the hormonal imbalance. I would be depressed if I couldn't budge my weight and couldn't control the hair growing on my body .

If you are in that category and have been told to go on a diet, swallow an antidepressant and get the hell out of anyone's surgery, get another opinion. If you feel that your hormones might be at the root of your low mood, keep looking for someone who gets it. Focus on handling your hormones first before trying an antidepressant because we know that will be the best way to fix your mood.

# Are hormones making my migraines worse?

Migraines are debilitating and they make lots of people miserable. And often they're hormonal. Around 70 per cent of migraine sufferers are women, of whom 60 to 70 per cent say their migraines are affected by their menstrual cycles. The usual pattern is that as oestrogen levels hit their low point – just before or during the period, migraines ramp up. Most migraine sufferers find that their headaches disappear when they're pregnant and oestrogen levels are high. But that's not the full picture with oestrogen being the trigger and not the reliever in other women, especially when the oestrogen comes in the form of HRT or the pill.

## How to handle your hormones

### PLAN AHEAD
If you're lucky enough to have a regular cycle, you know when your migraines are due to come on. So about three days before they typically start, you can start taking a non steroidal anti-inflammatory medicine or NSAID, such as ibuprofen or naproxen at

the recommended dose. They're available over the counter – just follow the directions on the packet. To work out which day to start, keep a headache journal for a couple of months or just start on day 19 of your cycle.

###### REGULAR EXERCISE
Just 30 minutes of aerobic exercise a day has been linked to less frequent and less severe migraines, hormonal or not.

###### MIGRAINE MEDICINES
If these strategies don't work, see your GP. There are a number of specific migraine preventers and treaters on the market in tablet form that in my experience work for most women.

## Stress and your hormones

Stress has a number of well documented effects on the mind and body. The whole purpose of your body's stress responses is to enable your mind and body to act quickly and forcefully if there is a threat. So for example the stress response includes stimulating the nerves of the brain to enable you to be vigilant and focused as well as inhibition of nerves in charge of non-vital functions, like eating, growth and reproduction. Your body changes to allow better oxygen supplies and nutrition to the brain, heart and muscles, which might be needed for a fight or flight response.

Feeling stressed often makes your memory go to water. We've worked out why. Short term cortisol boosts can actually sharpen your memory, as a great stress management tool. But long-term exposure to high cortisol levels harms the very brain cells it was intended to protect, especially those cells in the hippocampus. It's a kind of overuse injury. The hippocampus can't continually be hyperactive. It gets worn out. So to protect itself from burnout, the cells of the hippocampus simply reduce their connections to each other to counter the overstimulation. Ultimately the whole hippocampus shrinks and functions in a less efficient way. That's been proven.

There have actually been studies that have taken large groups of people and had them record on a daily basis how stressed they felt. The stress could be anything from financial worries, stress at work, stress about relationships or bad health etc. Then they also had their cortisol blood levels measured, their memory tested and the volume of the memory-storing hippocampus in the brain measured by MRI.

Consistently, people who report the highest levels of stress over a protracted period of time also have the highest blood levels of cortisol and people who report the least amount of stress have the lowest blood levels of cortisol. The people with that chronic stress and high cortisol had smaller hippocampi on MRI and did worse on their memory tests. And you guessed it; the low stress people with lower cortisol levels had larger hippocampi and did better at the memory tests. In case the reporting on stress and your brain is making you stressed, there's good news. We know that as stress goes away, your blood cortisol levels also decline, the size of your hippocampus increases again and the results of your memory tests go back to normal. Isn't the brain amazing?

# How to handle your stress hormones

### GET ORGANIZED, ESPECIALLY IF YOU'RE A STRESS HEAD ANYWAY

So there was a study that fascinated me and helps prove that the chicken (personality) came before the egg (mood!) This study looked at the personality traits of neuroticism (tending towards having negative or unstable moods and higher stress levels) and conscientiousness (the tendency to be organised, thorough and reliable) and linked them with the blood cortisol levels over a few days. Then it also linked daily mood swings with cortisol levels and how those same traits of neuroticism and conscientiousness affected this relationship.

The scientists found a linear link between neuroticism and the daily cortisol levels. In other words, the higher the neuroticism personality scores, the higher the cortisol production in general. Now, in this study conscientiousness did not decrease daily cortisol production directly but there was a linear relationship between conscientiousness and mood over time. The more conscientious someone was, the more stable their moods, the less frequent their bad mood days and the more frequent their good mood days.

And overall the authors found that people who reported that

they were having a good mood day produced less cortisol and on the flip side they had higher cortisol levels when they said they were in a worse mood. But it was the people who had the highest scores in conscientiousness who had the biggest reductions in cortisol when they were in a good mood.

Given that high cortisol levels are linked to immune system problems, anxiety, heart disease and diabetes, you can see that simply being organized can not only make you feel less distressed but will protect us from the ravages of aging as well.

### BREAK IT DOWN

Sometimes the task at hand or the problems you face are so enormous you just feel overwhelmed by the sheer weight of it all. You just have to break it up into small, manageable components that you can tick off one day at a time and wait to deal with the big picture until you're a little stronger

### HAVE SOME MICRO BREAKS

We women are pretty good at planning our holidays. They might only come once a year and might just be a few days but we do take our holidays or as I like to call them, our 'macro breaks' seriously. And we love them. And to round off the macro breaks we are not bad at arranging 'mini breaks'. These are your weekends away at a friend's farm or visiting Nan in the country. But these breaks, as wonderful as they are can be stressful to plan and their relaxing effect can disappear within days of returning home.

What we often miss is 'micro breaks' or the opportunity to take time out in the middle of a busy day. It might be just ten seconds you take out from your crazy schedule to STOP doing, running, thinking and just declutter your head for a moment or two. Close your eyes, take three or four deep breaths and start again. If you're waiting in the supermarket queue from hell, stuck in a traffic nightmare or being kept waiting by someone for a meeting or appointment, instead of letting the STRESS of doing nothing lead you to blow a gasket, let the peace of doing nothing recharge your batteries.

## DOWNLOADING TIME

Women spend all day uploading like maniacs, without properly filing the clutter inside our brains. You need to allocate some time to think to just get the hurricane in your head sorted. I recommend you combine this with exercise as the two just go hand in hand. One thing that happens when you go on a nice long solitary walk or run or swim is that your head just zones out. All of a sudden your brain stops uploading and BAM!! There's a window of opportunity and you end up downloading – like it or no. If you don't control your downloading time, it will control you at a time you really don't want it. Like at three am. All of a sudden you will wake up and remember the gas bill or the fact that your friend, Anne sounded a little strange on the phone yesterday. Maybe she's upset with you for some reason...Give your brain the space and time to sort this stuff out

## MINDFULNESS

I find this about the best stress buster going. It essentially gets you to be in the present and not to worry obsessively about what might be or was. Let me explain what I mean; look around the room and note down silently everything that is blue. Now close your eyes and recite them back to yourself. Without opening your eyes list the green things in the room. Best you're struggling to name more than one or two. You were so intent on studying the blue objects that the green objects simply escaped your attention. The mind is like that. Some of the cutest, funniest, loveliest, saddest and weirdest things can completely pass us by because we're so focused on the tasks in front of us.

One of the techniques used by psychologists dealing with people who are stressed, anxious or depressed is mindfulness. When you can't see a large picture of tranquillity and happiness, put one together with tiny patches of happiness from your day. But you need to notice them and take them on board. The feeling of the sun on your face when it's shining, the sound of children laughing, the smell of a fantastic coffee or a cake store, the look on your toddler's face when he stands on sand or laughs at Dora or Elmo. Those tiny moments can pass us by so quickly barely penetrating the surface of your busy, crazy, stressed out worlds. Don't let even one fly past without seizing it and making sure it sinks into your soul and adds a patch to your happiness quilt.

Similarly bad feelings, thoughts and experiences can sink in and grip into our soul like fishing hooks. Bad thoughts and feelings are arsenic for your soul. When a bad thought comes, allow it to emerge and then let it float away. Don't hold onto it, just imagine, like a leaf floating down a river that the thoughts pass through you instead of hooking into you. If you hold onto bad thoughts, they can really damage you.

## FORGIVENESS

Last week one of my beautiful patients came in to see me and she seemed really down. It turned out that well meaning friends and family members had been telling her they were pretty sure her ex husband was actually gay. She felt humiliated and deceived. After 15 years of marriage to hear this had left her angry, confused and hurt. What did that mean about her? "I just have to know" she said. She planned to confront him with these rumours and "get him to admit it to my face".

I could see what this was doing to her. We chatted for a bit and I asked her why she needed to know. How would it change her life? It didn't change the fact that they had experienced a very happy marriage for many years and that they shared beautiful children.

He had his own journey, his own life and he had to make peace with his demons. And she has to nourish her soul and live the best possible life she can. That means not miring her mind with negative and distressing, cortisol-inducing thoughts which will take their greatest toll on her.

Forgiveness is about YOU being able to let those destructive negative thoughts go, and not about condoning the behaviour of whoever has treated you badly. In so many cases, that person is getting on with their life and not giving you so much as a backward glance. The only one suffering is you. Let that negative energy go and with it, regain your sense of self and become the more positive, optimistic person you deserve to be.

I always refer to that sort of hurt and negativity as the dog poo you tread in by accident. Stepping in it in the first place is a nightmare. But it's happened. Now it's up to you. You can either wipe it off your shoe or continue to tread it through your house and ruin your carpets. In life the negativity you feel towards someone who has wronged you can be trod through your life like that dog poo. Without realising it, it can stop you from being able to get on with your life. Time to wipe that poo off your shoe and let it go. You don't have to be naive. You don't have to resume a friendship with someone who doesn't deserve it, but you can be free.

### GRATITUDE

It is so easy to spend your energy (and raise your cortisol levels) over things that are bad; things your friend has but that you can't afford, job success your colleague has had that has escaped you. But those feelings wreak havoc on your mind and body. It's time to focus on the good things that you have and the reasons you are fortunate. If you are feeling stressed or a little down, I want you right now to grab a pen and some paper and write down the first 10 things for which you are grateful that come into your head. I want you to include things you struggle with; your parents-in-law if they drive you crazy (they might have bought you something or looked after the kids when you were in a jam), your boss, even your husband. Whoever you feel is stressing you out a bit at the moment. Studies have found that being grateful is one of the most successful strategies to achieve real contentment and happiness. Try volunteering with people who are less fortunate than you for a real gratitude kick!

### SURROUND YOURSELF WITH GOOD ENERGY

One huge study that ran for twenty years confirmed what we have suspected for years; that being happy and content is contagious and sad sacks gravitate towards each other. It's obvious. Happy people are great to be around and make you enjoy yourself.

Lots of us have people in our lives whose bad energy brings us down. The phone number you dread seeing on your phone, the person with whom a visit is a chore. If those people are in your family, or are good friends going through a temporary hard time, you have to grin and bear it. But make your exposure as quick as possible and reward yourself by seeing a fun friend straight after to detox those negative vibes.

### Good music

Music is a perennial cultural de-stressor. If you are feeling uptight, a soft, rhythmic melody can really help bring you some inner peace. Studies have linked relaxing music with lower cortisol levels and less pain after an operation. The stress your body goes through when faced with an operation is not dissimilar to the everyday stress you have when work is tough or you have financial difficulties so it's a good comparison. So you can see how switching on the Adele playlist might work for you after the day from hell at work! Similar findings have emerged from studies of people who play an instrument themselves. Maybe best done in an empty house unless you're seriously talented. For me, picking up the guitar is like an instant distressing activity, even if it means stress for those poor family members who have to listen to me play. I can tell you our little one's recorder practice is like nails on a chalk board and I'd hate to take the rest of the family's cortisol levels after a recorder session!

### Green thumbs

Studies in both hospitals and in work places have shown that pot plants reduce stress and anxiety and increase productivity. I see a house with 1,000 little pots of African violets and half watered droopy Spathiphylla and I start to hyperventilate, but nice looking, and well maintained greenery does wonders for the soul. Scientists have identified substances called volatile organic compounds. These are the sorts of toxic chemicals that have become a part of our daily life as we are surrounded by plastic and chemicals. Pot plants have been shown to reduce levels of those toxic chemicals in a room. Maybe it's the lower toxic chemicals or perhaps it is the calming colour green. Either way, when your house feels like a study in madness, a little pot plant action is the way to go.

And you could possibly take it one step further; in one Dutch study, two groups of people were given a stressful task and afterwards they either read indoors or did some gardening for 30 minutes. Afterward, the group that gardened reported being in a better mood than the reading group, and they also had lower levels of the cortisol. So if you do have a plot of dirt, get your fingers dirty and plant away

### AROMATHERAPY

In a nice little double-blind placebo-controlled study of menopausal women with mood swings, a combination of bergamot, geranium, lavender and clary sage inhaled from a bottle for two minutes three times a day for five days significantly helped women with mood swings compared to a placebo blend. They reported feeling less moody and there was also a drop in their salivary cortisol levels. But lots of lovely essential oils have been used by aromatherapists for years to help with stress and anxiety. Even without the nice randomized placebo controlled trial to back them up, they are certainly unlikely to do you any harm.

### CHEWING GUM

Ok this one sounds nutty right? But there was a cute study of 20 stressed out twenty and 30-somethings who were asked to perform some stressful tasks both chewing gum and then not chewing gum. Chewing gum made these study subjects significantly more alert and they reported less stress while doing their tasks. Plus they had lower levels of salivary cortisol. Plus apparently their tasks were performed better. I know what I will do next time a complex patient comes in for a tricky diagnosis!

### GET A PET

We know that sitting calmly and patting a dog lowers cortisol levels in a laboratory setting. I am guessing the same would apply to any pet (maybe not a pet python, but a rabbit or cat!) Pet therapy has been shown to be beneficial, especially for teenagers and for the elderly.

I'm biased because I just love my dogs. They make me laugh and I love how happy they get to see me when I come home from work. But if you live in an apartment or pet ownership is not an option for another reason, maybe get a pet fix at a local animal shelter or head to the local park and play ball with someone else's dog!

# Are My Hormones Destroying My Sex life?

When sex goes pear-shaped, hormones often cop the blame and they're often at the root of at least some of the issues that are stuffing up your sex life.

Sexual dysfunction, or problems, including low sex-drive, inability to achieve orgasm, vaginal dryness and painful sex are the sorts of problems I deal with in my practice and many of these problems do have a hormonal basis. These problems are so common and yet so rarely talked about. A US study estimated that up to 43 per cent of women have some level of sexual dysfunction and that the chances increase as you get older.

## Hormones and sex

In women, let's start with your female hormones. Oestrogen increases blood flow to you genitals, which has a couple of effects. Firstly, it basically maintains glands from the uterus and cervix as well as the Bartholin's glands that sit at the very bottom of the introitus (vaginal opening). These glands are charged with ensuring a steady supply of the vaginal lubrication that is constantly present but that increases after nerve stimulation that happens with sexual arousal. Then the vaginal walls themselves produce fluid, again under encouragement by oestrogen. As you can imagine, anything that decreases the amount of oestrogen in the vagina will decrease the amount of lubrication as well. Plus drier cells are more prone to getting traumatised during sex, so sex can be a bit painful if there's no oestrogen around. All this makes it harder to achieve an orgasm, right?

Androgens (male hormones) are also believed, but not proven, to be important for sexual function in women. Recent research has linked low libido to low testosterone levels in women.

Interestingly, in women, testosterone starts to drop off as early as your late 20s at a slow and steady rate until reaching about 50 per cent of their peak levels by the time you hit menopause.

## The physiology of sex

I think that as a woman, you should know what happens from the first sexy thought through to your orgasm. It's sciency, nerdy and incredibly unsexy. But it's also incredibly complex and it will give you an appreciation of why it's so easy for things to go wrong.

Not surprisingly, sexual arousal all starts in the brain. In response to a stimulus (a photo of George Clooney with his shirt off – am I showing my age? Maybe it's a look from your partner or a back massage) your hypothalamus, limbic system and hippocampus transmit nervous signals through both the parasympathetic and sympathetic nervous systems.

In response to the nervous stimulation, a cascade of chemicals is released from the nerves of the vagina, clitoris and vulva. An array of sexy sounding chemicals such as Neuropeptide Y, vasoactive intestinal polypeptide, nitric oxide synthase, cyclic guanosine monophosphate and substance P have been found in studies to exist in the vaginal nerve fibres, although exactly what role each plays is still unknown. The blood vessels supplying the clitoris, vagina and labia become engorged with blood and the vagina begins to secrete lubricating fluids. The uterine and Bartholin's glands also begin to provide lubrication for the vagina. The muscle walls of the vagina relax and the uterus sits higher in the pelvis and this is why the entire vagina both lengthens and widens to accommodate the enlarged penis heading its way. Meanwhile, stimulation of the clitoris also makes both its length and width increase and it becomes engorged with blood. But wait! There's more: increased muscle tension, causes erection of the nipples as well as tension in the arms and legs.

All of the swelling of the labia makes the labia minora or inner lips part, which makes the opening of the vagina more obvious. All the engorgement of the blood vessels in the genital area makes the labia and clitoris change colour, from skin colour to a pinkish colour. Once women have had children genitals can colour to a deeper red colour.

Ultimately with enough stimulation (which doesn't necessarily have to be genital by the way), you get your reward with major involuntary spasms of various muscle groups in the vagina and around the anus as well as a spike in heart rate and blood pressure. There's also increased activity in areas of the brain including the hypothalamus, midbrain, hippocampus and cerebellum. Hello orgasm!

During an orgasm your brain produces a large amount of oxytocin, which is at least responsible for the contractions on your uterus but which also make you feel closer to your partner and gives you that warm, stress-free, calm, happy feeling. We also know that both just before sex and just after sex, orgasm or no, your testosterone levels rise although what exactly that rise achieves, we're not sure. But you can imagine that a lack of testosterone would play some role in disrupting your sexual function.

So let's look at some of the hormonal conditions that can ruin your sex life, starting with the bleeding obvious:

# Is menopause wrecking my sex life?

Sexual problems are among the most common side effects of menopause. For a start, having a dry vagina won't help. Oestrogen keeps your vaginal cells moist and plump and robust, too. They're less prone to tearing and trauma during sex. So without oestrogen on board sex can be dry and painful and you can actually get little painful tears in the vagina. It's called vaginal atrophy and a lot of women don't talk about it. I tend to notice it while doing a pap test. I often ask women how sex has been since the menopause. Some are actually fine, but others have had to say Sayonara to their sex life because it is simply too uncomfortable. What a waste

If you head back to the Hormone Primer, don't forget that not only do you lose lots of oestrogen after menopause but you also lose lots of your male androgens as well, as there are less androgen in general being produced by the adrenal glands. DHEA, the major precursor to testosterone is down to around 10 to 20 per cent of its peak levels by the time you hit 70. Plus you have the enzyme, aromatase busily converting testosterone to oestrogen in the ovaries as well as the fat cells. So all in all there is a net fall off of testosterone as you age. And, if you remember, the androgens also play a role in your arousal and your general satisfaction with sex.

So if we accept that there is going to be a natural fall off of hormones responsible for arousal, orgasm, and libido, when do you have a problem?

# Hypoactive sexual desire disorder (HSDD)

HSDD is defined by the presence of two symptoms happening together:

* Persistent or recurrent deficiency (or absence) of sexual fantasies, thoughts, and/or desire for, or receptivity to, sexual activity and
* Personal distress caused by the sexual dysfunction described in the first criterion (that's YOUR distress not your husband's).

I read that and instinctively I thought it wouldn't be a huge number of women. So wrong! One study (admittedly set in a women's gynaecological clinic!) found that up to 50 per cent of all women meet the criteria for a diagnosis of HSDD!! While hormones play a huge role in theory, they seem to only play a small role in practice. A large study compared hormone levels and HSDD symptoms and found there was very little correlation between the two.

We know that women with a blood DHEA level in the bottom 10th centile are more likely to have sexual problems. But because women with low DHEA won't necessarily have HSDD or any other sexual dysfunction, obviously there's more to the problem than just hormonal issues. We think that the DHEA might just be a symptom of something else going on as opposed to the cause of the problems. For example, we know that stress and chronic disease can lower your DHEA levels and also tend to wipe out your libido and sexual function in general.

There are some women with genuine low androgen levels. For example, women who have had their ovaries removed because of cancer or severe endometriosis often have a lot of problems due to low testosterone. But for the rest of us, hormones might only be a part of the problem...

So given that, what do you do if your sex life is in the doldrums?

## How to handle your hormones

Here are some things that are REALLY worth a shot

### Get enough sleep

In my practice, because I see so many mums with little children, peri-menopausal women, and women who are just so ridiculously busy, they don't have enough hours in the day; sleep deprivation is almost the norm. While these women feel exhausted and are aware of the general brain fug, they often don't put two and two together and associate the quantity and quality of their rapidly declining sex life with their lack of Zzzzs.

Sleep deprivation has a few effects on your sex life. First of all, your hottest bedroom fantasy involves a pillow and gentle snore. Sleep will trump sex in any position. In a contest between the ten or twenty minutes to achieve orgasm and slipping exhausted into dreamland, your orgasm doesn't stand a chance.

Next is the fact that when you're sleep deprived, all those semi-foreplay activities like going out for dinner in a sexy dress are off the agenda. A survey by the National Sleep Foundation in 2009 found that insomniacs are three times more likely to skip 'social activities' because they're tired.

Thirdly, sleep deprivation wreaks havoc with your relationships. You are more likely to snap at your partner, be critical, annoyed, frustrated and less likely to notice how cute he looks in that new shirt! (See below for some tips on fixing the relationship)

### GET SOME EXERCISE

This is one of the best interventions for sexual problems around. Countless studies have actually looked at this. Without a doubt people who regularly work out have more sex, and enjoy sex more. When you tease out the exact link between regular exercise and sex, we know that higher physical endurance and more muscle tone both independently improve your sex life. Perhaps it is the endorphins released after a vigorous workout that kick your sex life along. In one recent study, women were more sexually responsive following 20 minutes of vigorous exercise than after no exercise at all.

And a nice little study on rats proved that after exercise, more testosterone is converted to the more potent dihydrotestosterone or DHT form straight after exercise.

Then again, I suspect that statistically, women who work out are more likely to have the sorts of bodies that favour lights on nudity than couch potatoes. Feeling flabby and unattractive won't put too many of us in the mood.

Plus, we know regular exercise has a powerful effect on your mood and in turn, low mood and low sexual function are regular bedfellows. Excuse the dad joke.

Whatever the link, the jury is in! Do more exercise and not only will you boost your mood, lose weight, prevent and manage chronic diseases and sleep better but we will throw in a better sex life for free!

### GET YOUR MEDICAL PROBLEMS SORTED

Medical problems can definitely affect your libido. Whether you have a sore hip from arthritis, which makes half the sexual positions an adventure in agony, or whether you're so tired from breathlessness that anything other than sitting still on a chair leaves you exhausted, unmanaged diseases need to get sorted out. See your GP and discuss the impact of the conditions you have on your sex life and see whether their management can be tweaked a little.

If you don't have any obvious medical problems, you should still get checked for low iron and underactive thyroid. Both of these conditions are so easy to diagnose and fix (either with iron replacement therapy or thyroid replacement therapy) and if that's all that stands between you and a killer sex life, you're laughing!

### GET SOME COUNSELLING

Sexual counseling is a curious area. It really does attract some strange types! It is also an area that tends to be pretty poorly regulated. I can't tell you how to find a good sex therapist, but in my experience, for couples who are keen on exploring tantra and the use of sex toys with a sex therapist, they're doing pretty well and probably don't need one.

The sort of therapy I'm talking about of course is couples counseling but with someone who is well equipped to discuss the intricacies of your physical relationship as well. Someone who can integrate the physical, the spiritual and the emotional aspects of your love life.

I asked my friend Dr Nikki Goldstein, who is an amazing sexologist, how to find a decent counsellor in this tricky space. Here is her advice:

"When it comes to finding a sex therapist, it's like finding a lid to fit on your pot, they are all so different and have a different way of treating people. The first thing would be to look at your potential counsellor's qualifications but not necessarily knock someone back who isn't heavily qualified. There are so many ways to tackle issues to do with sex and sometimes those that come from a more holistic and spiritual background can be just as much if not more effective than those who come from an academic one.

Read through what type of therapies and specialties they have. Most therapists these days do have websites. You also don't have the pressure of continuing with a therapist you are not sure about and you can be honest with wanting a first meeting to see if there is a good fit. Don't see the first session as a therapeutic session as such but rather a trial to see if you feel comfortable with them and also to ask questions about their process and how they treat their clients. If you do not feel there is a good fit don't be ashamed to discuss this with the therapist and ask them if they can refer you to someone who might fit a specific category you are looking for."

### STRENGTHEN YOUR PELVIC MUSCLES

They're the bane of the pregnant woman. We are all constantly reminded to do our pelvic floor (or Kegel) exercises. Well it turns out that doing so will not only prevent you from having a little overflow accident every time you cough or run for the bus, but pelvic floor exercises can also make sex more enjoyable and increase your libido. To perform these exercises, tighten your pelvic muscles as if you're stopping a stream of urine. Hold for a count of five, relax and repeat. Do these exercises several times a day.

### VAGINAL OESTROGEN

If vaginal atrophy is your only menopausal issue, you don't need to resort to HRT, but you can put a tiny amount of oestrogen directly into the vagina to thicken and moisten the cells. The tiny amount is mostly absorbed directly into the vaginal cells and very little of it is absorbed into the blood stream so the risk of the sorts of side effects we had seen in the WHI study are not relevant here. Another advantage of the low dose is that it doesn't need to be counteracted with progesterone.

Vaginal oestrogen creams or pessaries are used every night for two weeks to get started. Then it's simply used twice a week for so long as having a good functioning vagina is important to you. It usually helps a little with the urine infections and weak pelvic floor that come packaged up with menopause as well.

### HRT

Nobody would suggest that you go on Hormone replacement therapy for low libido or sexual problems alone, but if you are going to be on them for another reason, like aches and pains, mood swings or hot flashes, you may well will get a bit of a boost to your libido for the same price!

### SWITCH FROM HRT TO TIBOLONE

We met the medication, Tibolone in the chapter Are My Hormones Making Me Tired? It gets broken into a chemical that mimics some of the effects of oestrogen but not others. It's great for bones, great for hot flashes but most importantly, it is also partially broken down into testosterone. As we've seen above that's not the full story but enough studies have shown that Tibolone benefits libido that it is at least worth considering.

### STRESS CONTROL

Stress is like cyanide for your libido. When your head is consumed with worries and anxiety, it can be impossible to be able to think about sex or orgasms. If I had a simple straightforward stress-nuking formula, I promise I would give it to you, but I don't. I just think it's important to acknowledge the role that stress plays in taking out your libido and your ability to really get into sex the way you'd like to.

If you are going through a short-term stressful period, such as uncertainty about your role at work or a serious illness in a family member or friend, maybe you should make the link and then take the pressure off yourself. Hopefully the situation will settle down and your sexual appetite and enjoyment will return to normal with it.

But if you are facing a run of protracted stress from financial woes, serious relationship breakdown or illness, then that's a different story. Sure, your sex life is going to fall apart but so are your physical and mental health and your sleep. People under chronic stress are at risk of drug and alcohol issues and poor performance at work. There are so many reasons to tackle this issue. And to be honest, fixing your sex life is a pretty minor one!

The problem I find with so many of my patients is they don't really recognise it. They're so mired in the morass of stress that their lives have become that they can't see the effect it's having on them. If they could take a step back like I do – simply by being an impartial third party looking in at the situation, they would definitely want to do whatever it takes to feel better.

When it comes to stress, you can't look to blame others or change the situation you're in. It is all about you being able to manage the situation you're in better so that the same stressful events don't take such a massive toll on you. Whether you choose prayer and church, the comfort of close friends, rigorous exercise or meditation, it's up to you. And most people need to try a few different things to find something that works.

## MEDICATION REVIEW

If you take medications for medical problems, head to your GP or pharmacist for a medication review. So many really common medications cause sexual problems. For example, all sorts of blood pressure medicines such as Clonidine, Lisinopril and Metoprolol can interfere with both your libido and your ability to reach an orgasm. Ditto lots of the sleeping or anti-anxiety pills such as Diazepam, Alprazolam and Lorazepam. Being on regular cortisone for arthritis or asthma, for example, can also wreak havoc on your libido by suppressing your adrenal glands' ability to make DHEA and as a result depleting at least half of your available testosterone. In almost every case, there is an alternative that won't destroy your sex life, but you HAVE to raise the issue with your health professional because if they don't know it's bothering you, they're unlikely to bring up the option of switching medications.

## DETOX

I'm not talking wheatgrass and whacky restrictive diets. I'm talking about the anxiolytic in a bottle, the old wine o'clock. Alcohol hits sexual function pretty badly. I know what you're saying; a couple of champers to get you in the mood is definitely not a libido killer. I agree. It's the three or four wines you drink night in night out that takes the legs of your sex life out from under you. Apart from falling into a sleepy coma every night where the only chance you have of getting sex is if your partner is a fan of necrophilia, excess alcohol physically interferes with the complex sexual functioning of your body.

And if you're a fan of weed, or any other illicit drug, it is a serious culprit for sexual dysfunction. From marijuana to cocaine, ecstasy and amphetamines through to barbiturates and heroin, all are strongly implicated with sexual dysfunction. It's funny me advising you to ditch these habits for the benefit of your sex life. There is NO REASON to stay on this stuff. Dangerous, illegal, putting you at risk of criminal prosecution, expensive and potentially dirty, bad for your mood and your brain in general, to be honest restoring your sex life is pretty much the least important reason to get off this stuff. But I mention it because you might spend a lot of time and energy trying to get your libido sorted and that will be a complete waste if you keep rolling a joint semi regularly.

## LUBRICANTS

While we're waiting for vaginal oestrogen to kick in, in the case of menopause, or while we're waiting for your relationship to light up, lubricants can right a lot of short term wrongs. They certainly make sex less uncomfortable and take the pressure off you before the act so you don't have to worry about whether or not it will hurt and whether you will 'perform' on the night. There are specific vaginal lubricants on the market, as well as generic ones, like KY Jelly. My favourite? Saliva! Works a treat!!

Here are some things that MIGHT be worth a shot and won't harm you

## DHEA SUPPLEMENTS

We met the hormone, DHEA (dehydroepiandrosterone) in our hormone primer. But to refresh your memory, it is a hormone produced by the adrenal glands and is often referred to as the mother of hormones, because it is converted in the body to so many other hormones, including both oestrogen and testosterone. Your own natural levels of DHEA decline naturally with age. This process actually starts at age 20! Both low DHEA and low testosterone have been linked with low libido, which is why studies have examined whether DHEA supplements can boost libido.

Seven trials have been published that investigated the use of DHEA supplements for the treatment of low libido and low sexual function in otherwise healthy women. A benefit for sexual function was reported in only three out of the seven studies, and each of these three studies had some major flaws to the way they were conducted, making the conclusions less convincing from them. But in all seven, supplementing the women with DHEA increased levels of DHEA in the blood actually restoring levels to the so-called 'young levels'.

There are some things you should be aware of when taking DHEA. Firstly, there are some nasty side effects that have been reported including acne, male pattern hair growth, spare-tyre style weight gain around the middle, high blood pressure and lower levels of HDL (AKA "good" cholesterol). And because DHEA is converted to oestrogen and testosterone in the body, people with hormone sensitive cancers, especially breast, ovary and endometrial, should never take it.

Plus, high doses of DHEA might be toxic to the liver. Lastly, as there have been no long-term studies on the safety of DHEA, we can't put our heads on a block and tell you there are no risks. It interacts with lots of your medications. You're probably wondering why in this case, I have said it isn't dangerous? That's because, presuming you get it prescribed by a doctor, they will make sure they monitor you for any side effects and stop the supplement should any occur. However, there are potential issues if you get DHEA supplements yourself online. Obviously I think that is really stupid because you never know what's in anything you buy online and with something so potentially dangerous, I would only ever go to a trusted source and have medical supervision.

### Look after the skin on your lady bits

I see lots and lots of women who are spending vast sums of money at the local pharmacy after having diagnosed themselves with a yeast infection. Hint – if the burning and itching isn't getting better, yeast may not be the issue! I see so much eczema and dermatitis where the sun don't shine, you would be amazed! If you have a red, swollen, sore vulva, you need help! Firstly, never EVER use soap down there. It has a very high pH which will not only dry out the skin horribly but will raise the risk of infections such as thrush. Use a pH neutral cleanser or simple sorbelene. You will also probably need a prescription cortisone cream to decrease the inflammation. Until it has resolved, no penis vagina penetrative sex! Doctor's orders!!

### Ginkgo biloba

This ancient Chinese herb, used for centuries in traditional Chinese medicine, has been purported to cure everything from dementia and the cognitive impairment of dementia to circulatory problems. In North America, it is most commonly used to improve cognitive function and memory in people with age-related cognitive decline and memory loss. But when it comes to low libido and sexual dysfunction, many of the studies to date have had pretty woeful results, suggesting it is no better than a placebo. There was one interesting study, though of 33 men and women with depression and low libido. After taking 40 or 60 mg twice daily of *ginkgo biloba* extract for four weeks, 91 per cent of women and 76 per cent of men reported that they had improvements in desire, 'arousal' (erection and lubrication) and orgasm. But there was no 'control' arm, so we can't conclude too much. A subsequent placebo-controlled trial of 99 women with sexual dysfunction found that both placebo and *ginkgo biloba* helped with sexual problems. But in that study, the placebo achieved slightly higher success than the *ginkgo*! Kinda makes you wonder about the power of the placebo effect. Either way, it was a bigger, better study suggesting ginkgo was at best no better than a placebo.

And there are potential problems with ginkgo, too. Apart from minor problems like nausea, headache, dizziness and allergic skin reactions, it can interfere with fertility, with the sugar control of your diabetes and with your ability to make blood clots. Chat to your GP before starting ginkgo.

SELEGILINE

This is a drug for Parkinson's disease and depression. That's because it blocks the actions of an enzyme in the brain called mono amine which breaks down feel-good neurotransmitters including dopamine, serotonin and melatonin. During studies for Parkinson's Disease, an increase in libido was found to be a major side effect in some people, which got people thinking about using it for exactly that purpose! So today lots of doctors use it in very low doses to give your libido a kick. We don't have good trial data to suggest it's useful but then again, the studies haven't been done and we don't know that it's not useful either. The dose in your 50s is 5 mg Mon through Friday, in your 60s it is five mg six times a week and in your 70s, it's taken every day. For women in their 40s it is taken on Mondays, Wednesdays and Fridays.

It isn't without side effects though. There are some minor irritations, like dizziness, dry mouth, insomnia and muscle pains and it can also give you an abnormal heart rhythm. Talk it through with your doctor. This is growing in popularity in the USA and it's certainly got its devotees even though the jury is still out on its effectiveness.

### L-ARGININE SUPPLEMENTS

L-arginine is an amino acid (protein building block) that your body uses to make nitric oxide, a chemical that helps to relax blood vessels and allow blood to flow through arteries. Studies on L-arginine supplements for sexual dysfunction in women have used a combination product with pycnogenol, which makes it impossible to know if any improvement was due to the L-arginine or other ingredients in the formula. But taking five grams per day may be effective.

It does have a couple of side effects though, such as lowering your blood pressure. Particularly if you use it with other medications used to lower blood pressure. There is also some concern, although not proven, that L-Arginine may make flare-ups of herpes virus worse as the virus itself needs this amino acid to replicate. For that reason, most doctors recommend people with recurrent herpes steer clear.

### SILDENAFIL (VIAGRA)

It's designed and marketed to men but increasingly, women are trying to get a bit of the Viagra action. This medication inhibits the enzyme, phosphodiesterase-5 (PDE5), which allows the smooth muscle in the walls of the arteries to relax, leading to greater blood flow, especially to the genitals. It peaks in the blood stream about an hour after you take it.

In an eight week placebo-controlled trial of 100 young women (average age 37) with sexual dysfunction from antidepressants, Sildenafil (either 50 or 100 mg before sexual intercourse) was twice as effective at improving libido and general sexual function as a placebo. There's no evidence that Sildenafil helps women who aren't on an anti-depressant and even the study that was done was too small to make firm conclusions. Plus, it was funded by the drug company that makes Viagra; however, it might be worth a shot. I have had some patients use it and report really good results, especially in the peri-menopausal era.

### ANTI-DEPRESSANTS

The whole Viagra thing brings up an interesting point. Between 30 and 70 per cent of people treated for major depression with an antidepressant end up with sexual problems. Sexual dysfunction is a well documented side effect of antidepressants. That is thought to be the major cause of what we call non-compliance, or basically chucking the tablets in a drawer and forgetting about them. I passionately believe in getting help for major depression. At its worst, moderate to severe major depression can be fatal, through suicide. And people suffering from depression have a higher risk of a raft of chronic diseases and early death.

But some people are experiencing negative side effects (not only sexual dysfunction but sometimes nausea, light- headedness and tremors as well) without need. If you have been on antidepressant medications for ages, you may no longer need them. Or if you have only mild to moderate depression or anxiety, you could do just as well with regular exercise, therapy with a counsellor or just *Hypericum* or St John's wort, which doesn't cause any sexual problems whatsoever. So have a chat to your GP about whether the benefits of the antidepressant medicines outweigh the chop to your libido.

### DAMIANA

Damiana (*Turnera diffusa*) is a herb used traditionally by the Mayan people of Central America to enhance sexual function in men and women. It is reported to be an aphrodisiac, stimulant, mood enhancer, and a tonic. The good news is it's safe and is unlikely to harm you. The bad news is there's no evidence whatsoever that it will give your libido anything like a boost despite its heavy promotion.

### YIN YANG HUO OR HORNY GOAT WEED (*EPIMEDIUM*)

There are a number of plants, weeds really of the *Epimedium* species that fall under that name. Legend has it that a Chinese goat herder noted that his goats started mating like crazy whenever they started grazing on this plant. It contains a flavonol called icariin, which WEAKLY inhibits the same enzyme, phosphodiesterase-5 (PDE5) as Sildenafil. Only Sildenafil is 80 times more potent than icariin in inhibiting phosphodiesterase-5. In fact, studies in bunnies show that you'd have to take an impossibly enormous amount of horny goat weed to get a mere tenth of the effectiveness of Sildenafil. And we have no studies in women. But there aren't any side effects and I'm impressed with the placebo effects given the number of patients who give me glowing reports despite the lack of scientific credibility.

### Sexy lingerie, waxing and more

Girls, if you want to feel sexy, be prepared to invest a little in your sex appeal. In my experience this is about YOU getting in the mood rather than looking acceptable to your partner. Surveys have found that what men find the most sexy thing about a bed partner is not her perky boobs or lack of cellulite, but her enthusiasm. He is generally OK with how you look, but making love with someone who clearly doesn't want to be there is not a massive turn on to him. We women on the other hand are often revolted by our appearance to the point where we just do not feel in the slightest bit sexy. So this is for you; let's try getting you into the swing of things by trying to feel a little sexier.

First step, off to the beautician. A little grooming from armpits and legs to your bikini line and beyond might be your thing. Might not be either. If you feel sexy with the fully untrimmed hedge, that's great!! Next step is to buy some sexy lingerie. I have not known too many women who don't feel sexier in a bit of negligee. Now if being sprung in that section of the underwear store by your daughter-in-law makes you feel nauseous, aren't we lucky to live in the online shopping era? The stuff available will blow your mind! From the prettiest, laciest, pinkest knickers to naughty nursemaids and everything in between, it's all there.

Lastly, a nice shower or bath with some smelly soaps, some smelly moisturisers, some smelly shampoo and conditioner, followed by a nice bit of lip gloss and you'll be ready to rock and roll. Or maybe just slightly less unready. It won't hurt anyway.

# What not to use for a flagging libido

### Yohimbe

The bark of the herb yohimbe (*Pausinystalia yohimbe*) was historically used as a folk remedy for sexual dysfunction. Not only have we found the herb to be ineffective for low libido and sexual dysfunction in women, it is potentially dangerous with severe side effects. It has been linked to mania, worsening of anxiety, irregular or rapid heartbeat, kidney failure, seizures, heart attack, and more. I don't recommend anyone take it.

### Testosterone Patches

Look, we've already discussed the fact that low testosterone doesn't necessarily equate that well with low sexual function. You can't really take testosterone as tablets because it gets rapidly destroyed after absorption. Studies have actually shown that an hour after a testosterone tablet, your levels go back to normal. That's why it tends to be worn as a patch and they're available all over the place, especially online without prescription.

There are two issues with testosterone patches. Firstly we have no long-term safety data for their use in women. Nobody can tell you that they don't carry risks because we do not know. Secondly there are some pretty nasty side effects, especially: greasy skin and hair, scalp itching, hair loss from your head, and lots of body hair (hirsutism). These are all effects of excess androgens. See Are My Hormones Making Me Look Bad?

# Getting the relationship sorted

Lots of my patients have fabulously happy partnerships. Years after the kids have started school, when many of their friends' marriages are getting stale, they're still happy with their soul mate. Others aren't as lucky. After the initial burning fire of passion, lust and idol worshipping has died down, they are often living with someone who they find less attractive inside and out.

Bottom line, many do love each other, but somehow the relationship which once consumed every waking moment has become their last priority. Their attention and effort goes to their kids, their friends, their work colleagues, even the local vegetable seller, but not their partner.

In turn they often feel unloved, uncared for, unsupported and unappreciated. It's hard to want to go down on someone who doesn't give you the time of day. So when it comes to fixing your sex life, it ain't going to happen without first fixing your relationship.

But you have to really work out that it's worth the effort. If you want to get your relationship back where it belongs, as a source of fun, comfort, happiness, calm, joy and orgasms in your life, then it's going to require some mental readjustment in your head and some hard work!

For a little mental readjustment, think about this; my HAPPY YOU formula.

### The best thing you can do for yourself and your children is have a happy partnership.

Just sit with that for a second. All of us take our relationship for granted. But have you thought about it from that perspective? Happy marriage = happy you = happy kids. I know that is very simplistic but being in a stale or even a terrible relationship full of anger (whether suppressed or expressed!) is stressful. And living with someone who loves, respects, understands you and wants what is best for you can make the good times better and the bad times less stressful.

If you're ready to commit to the concept of reprioritising your relationship up the scale of things that matter, I want you to write down your ten best memories as a couple and the ten things you like most about your partner. If you honestly cannot think of any good character traits and you have only four or five happy memories, you need to see a counsellor and decide whether this marriage is salvageable. But assuming you're relationship isn't a total train wreck, spend some time thinking about the good in your partner and why you committed to him in the first place.

The next step is getting out of your corner and acknowledging that to make things better will involve effort on BOTH parts. I have spent so much time with my patients who can list their top 20 reasons why their husband is a shit. They almost never talk about the role they play in the relationship that has gone sour. Nobody is perfect and coming up with a list of demands of things HE needs to change is not a reasonable strategy to move forward. There is always room for improvement and you need to get ready to do some cleaning up in your own backyard at the same time as asking for some effort from him.

The third step is sorting out your communication.

Why is it that after a while, our communication goes to pot

and we say things we don't mean and don't say the things we do mean? Here is this person you decided to make a life with. Because he was the one you liked most of all, because you wanted to commit to being exclusively with each other, maybe because you wanted to have a family together and because you wanted to grow old together. Now, even for the vast majority of my patients who are really committed to their significant relationships, their partner is copping the worst of their mouth.

So, having decided that this is the most significant relationship of your life and the one which has the greatest potential impact on your happiness and wellbeing, you need to put it on a pedestal. That means not just letting rip when you're annoyed but holding it all back for the teacher at the local school. Your partner needs the best of you. It means telling him how much he means to you, that you're really happy things are going well at work and that you can't wait for the weekend when you get a babysitter and have some time without the kids. It means telling him in a collaborative and mature way if something he does and says hurts or upsets you and not yelling exaggerated or nasty insults at him. It means sharing responsibility for making the relationship work and for tackling the things that don't work together.

Get that right and you mightn't even need sex counselling, lubricants or expensive supplements from the health food shop. Get that right and having sex might be something you look forward to, not dread.

Sold? Brilliant! So now having decided to put the toe back into the sexy water, where do you start?

# Where do I start?

When your sex life has been on hold or effectively absent for a while, the thought of going there again isn't exactly like riding a bike. It takes time and patience and often a gritty determination to make it work. Here are my top tips:

PLANNING
How unbelievably unromantic! Spontaneity may not be appropriate during the early days. What with your extensive grooming regimen and perhaps a few candles and a sexy playlist for your

iPod, you have to get organised right? You want to have done your exercise, been to the GP and changed around all your medications and ensured any little children are down for the count for the evening. You also do not want to initiate sex at 11 pm when you have a 6 am wake-up call and you've been at work all day. Because your idea of great sex at this hour will be the quickest wham bam thank you ma'am you can manage so you can get to sleep ASAP. NOT the ideal way to enjoy the experience.

### Try non-sexual intimacy
If sex isn't working take the pressure off. Tell your husband you want a night of intimacy instead and if it ends in sex, fantastic. If it doesn't, would you be freaked out if he masturbated in front of you to close the loop? Start with massages, kissing, stroking and touching. See how you feel.

### Massage therapy
There are people who do not like to be massaged. I have personally met them. I don't necessarily understand them but I promise they exist. For the rest of us, having a neck or back massage can become erotic so easily. The initial non sexual massage makes you relax. Perhaps add some massage oils with essential oils like lavender for relaxation. Now add some music. Some people like pan pipes and whale love songs but I honestly don't care whether it's ACDC as long as it relaxes you. Indeed studies have found that a simple non-intimate oil-free massage alone can lower cortisol levels by 31 per cent while increasing feel-good serotonin levels by 28 per cent and dopamine levels by 31 per cent. Whether you are giving or receiving, focusing on the touch, the smell or the sounds can put you in the mood.

### Start with the lights off
After taking a break for a while (from sex altogether or from decent sex!), you will want to walk before you run. There is plenty of time to grab the *Karma Sutra* and try the positions play book in your naughty nurse outfit and handcuffs, but let's just start by making the whole thing as unthreatening as possible. That means removing anything that will make you self conscious about the size of your butt!!

Once again, my friend and guru in all matters sex, Dr Nikki Goldstein has some brilliant advice to add:

Dr Nikki's top tips on rebooting your love life when it's gone stale:

* I think the first and most important thing to tell yourself is that this (stale sex life) is normal. We are not meant to stay in the honeymoon period of our sexual relationships forever and for some people it can be worse than for others. But that is OK, and you need to keep repeating that to yourself over and over again. It is also a process and one that is different for each and every person. You need to see your relationship as independent to everyone else's and not get caught up in comparisons of normality. There is no such thing as normal when it comes to sex!

  You need to first of all take the pressure off each other because it's not necessarily a lack of sex that can harm a relationships but the pressure that people put on each other during this time. Enjoy the time together exploring and communicating and be supporting and caring to each other, not stressful and angry.

* Before you even think about intercourse, it's important to address the relationship and the intimacy you share or maybe do not share at this stage. Communication is going to be your best tool in the battle to get things back on track. You need to make sure you have this down pat and that you know how to talk to your partner about the more delicate issues surrounding sex. My biggest hint for this is to try and take any heated emotions out of the conversation and always compliment your partner and reassure them of your love before you might deliver a statement that is criticising. When it comes to the intimacy side of things you need to make sure that you are able to switch off from the outside world and reconnect with each other. This might take some sessions of just being together without any interruptions, talking about your day, your dreams or what's on your mind. Sharing your inner most thoughts with your partner has the ability to bring you closer and also give them an idea of what is going on in your head.

* Scheduling sexy time is another great tip for intimacy. When you are busy you need to see working on your relationship as a priority. I advise scheduling time in each week just to be together with the possibility of maybe something more happening – but definitely no pressure.
* Once you have taken off the pressure and worked on communication and intimacy, it is time for something a little more physical. Before you reach for your whips and chains after reading *50 Shades of Grey*, it does not have to be that much of a drastic change or that hard core. It's important to look at one thing at a time and if you are into something more extreme, do your research and build towards it.

One small change will do for now. It can be something basic like a blindfold or massage oil. The important thing here is to change things slightly and see how your partner responds. It's also about trial and error. You need to find things that both people will enjoy and be careful not to cross someone's boundaries.

Great advice!

# Are my hormones giving me breast pain?

This is one of the commonest problems I see in general practice. Talk about a sure-fire way to kill off your sex life! Having your breasts feel like they're about to pop out of your chest, and thinking that if anyone touches them you will poke his eyes out with a fork, is not going to set your sex life on fire!

Breast pain is super common. Studies have found that 30 per cent of premenstrual women suffer breast pain for more than five days a month, badly enough to interfere with sexual, physical, social and work-related activities. And one study found that of women attending a clinic for breast cancer screening (so we're talking 40 plus women here), 69 per cent had breast pain. Studies find that the stress levels of these women with severe breast pain are as high as those in women with breast cancer about to have an operation.

It's oestrogen that really drives breast growth. Breast tissue has lots of oestrogen receptors, especially in the ducts and glands. On the other hand, progesterone seems to turbo-charge the growth of the rest of the breast tissue. If you think of the menstrual cycle as a dress rehearsal for pregnancy, it makes sense that in the second half of the cycle, the luteal phase, the breasts are getting prepared for pregnancy and breastfeeding a newborn. That's why everything is growing and expanding under the influence of all the oestrogen and progesterone being pumped out of the corpus luteum in the ovary.

Lots of my patients tell me that their breast pain and tenderness starts accelerating once they hit their 40s. No longer needing this breast tissue with which to feed a newborn, it is incredibly ironic that from the day of ovulation, simply turning over in bed without a bra can be pretty damned agonising. Some experts think that the relationship works like this: the breasts of women in their 40s have gone through so many extra menstrual cycles than younger women. As a result these women have more developed, more mature breast tissue with a greater number of breast tissue cells than younger women. And these cells are now programmed to grow like mad in response to the usual hormonal stimulation of your cyclical roller coaster. It's a theory that makes sense to me. Another theory that makes sense is that the breast pain is due to oestrogen dominance instead of progesterone in the second half of your cycle because you're either not ovulating any more or your corpus luteum doesn't function as well so doesn't make enough progesterone in the luteal phase. Finally, there's a belief that the breast pain comes from higher prolactin levels.

In my patients, especially those over 40, I do order a mammogram and ultrasound just to be on the safe side. After all, one in nine women does get breast cancer. Based on statistics alone, some women who have hormonal breast pain will have breast cancer, even if the two aren't necessarily connected. In fact breast pain, while it definitely CAN be a symptom of breast cancer, isn't a common one. I'm going to assume now that you've had your tests and that there's nothing treatable found on the mammogram or ultrasound.

# How to handle your hormones

### RELAX AND WAIT UNTIL MENOPAUSE

With hormonal breast pain that comes on before the period, it WILL settle down once your menopause is over. For many of my patients, knowing it's just a normal thing that happens as you get older is enough. Indeed studies do show that for 85 per cent of women, knowing there's nothing wrong with their breasts is all they need.

### GET A DECENT BRA

Look, this just makes sense, even if there weren't two small pro-spective studies which concluded just that. In the studies, women who wore an individually fitted bra or a sports bra experienced a 75 to 85 per cent improvement in breast pain. So go get yourself fitted for a new bra because it is obviously going to help.

### SMALL DOSE OF DIURETIC

Breast pain is made much worse under the careful watch of the progesterone in the second half of your cycle. A small dose of frusemide (20 mg first thing in the morning) or spironolactone (25 mg first thing) will often reduce the pain substantially, and for the same price will throw in less ankle swelling and less tight rings on your fingers! You can increase the dose to 40 mg of frusemide in the morning if the lower dose doesn't work. But you will need a prescription from your doctor and beware! Taking a diuretic means you will need ready access to a toilet for the extra pee in the morning! I have to point out here that despite the fact that this treatment is really successful for my patients (it often gets rid of the problem altogether), there's no trial data to support it.

### SWITCH TO TIBOLONE

We just saw tibolone's role in tackling low libido, but studies have found it causes less breast pain than HRT for menopause. If you get breast pain from HRT, chat to your doctor about switching over to tibolone.

### CHASTE BERRY (*VITEX AGNUS CASTUS*)

Chaste berry is believed to work by suppressing the release of prolactin from the pituitary gland. I love this one and frequently recommend it to my patients, especially if they suffer from pre-menstrual syndrome or PMS in general. There was a great little double-blind, placebo controlled trial of 104 women which pitted chaste berry capsules or liquid against placebo for at least three menstrual cycles. There was a statistically significant reduction in breast pain for the women having chaste berry compared to those who took a placebo.

Another double-blind, placebo-controlled study of 178 wom-en, looked at chaste berry for PMS in general. Again after three months, the women taking the chaste berry reported less breast tenderness as well as other PMS symptoms. There have been more trials showing the same results. These trials are small but they were well done trials and I certainly find it works with my patients.

You have to take it every day, not just before your period ,and the best dose is 20 mg taken one to three times daily. Start once a day and build up if you don't find it working. There are no side effects to worry about either.

### Flaxseed, linseed

There was one Canadian study that looked at the effects of flax-seed in women with severe cyclical breast pain. It took 116 women and put them through a double-blind placebo-controlled trial of either 25 grams of flaxseed daily (the seeds not the oil!), in a muf-fin, or a placebo muffin and then followed them for four menstru-al cycles. Interestingly all the women said they had less breast pain (that placebo effect again), but the women who were eating flaxseed had much more relief.

Getting flaxseed into your diet can be tough. The oil goes rancid and seriously disgusting really quickly. And while there is a reasonable amount in soy and linseed bread (flaxseed IS lin-seed), how do you know how much? You can buy linseeds and if you're up for measuring out 25 grams a day and chucking them on your breakfast cereal or on your salad, it wouldn't hurt at all.

### Vitamin E

There are five studies that have tackled the question of whether, and how Vitamin E helps breast pain or breast cysts. The three best quality studies (best because they were all randomised, double-blinded, placebo-controlled) found Vitamin E didn't work at all for breast pain or cysts. Then again, another two studies, but of poorer quality found it helped. Admittedly, in those trials, there really was only a tiny amount of symptom relief but it did help!

The problem is that some studies suggest high doses of vitamin E (>400 IU/day) could be linked to higher risk of death from any cause. On that basis I would suggest trying other treatments first.

### Evening primrose oil

I've included this because it is so popular. Studies have been done on evening primrose oil for breast pain with really disappointing results. Basically, at best it is a placebo. Having said that it is a pretty safe supplement and if you want to take it, feel free.

## What NOT to do about breast pain

### Ditch your coffee

No study has found any benefit from ditching coffee, despite the fact that you will read that and be told that almost everywhere. Coffee is so good for you! For a start, there's the ENORMOUS prospective study to date, published in the *New England Journal of Medicine*, which followed 229,119 men and 173,141 women over a period of 14 years and found that women who drank six cups of coffee a day were 15 per cent less likely to die – of anything – over the course of the study- than women who drank no coffee. There's also a benefit in terms of diabetes prevention with a huge meta-analysis of studies showing a seven per cent less risk of getting diabetes for every cup of coffee consumed each day. Coffee also reduces your risk of breast cancer, depression, Parkinson's disease, Alzheimer's disease, liver cancer and skin cancer. Plus it tastes so good! So don't give that up for something that won't work.

# Are My Hormones Making Me Look Bad?

Whether it's zits or random hairs in no place good, thinning of your mane or wrinkles, pigmentation or cellulite, your hormones are often at the core of what's making you feel bad about your appearance. In this chapter we will go through some of the less attractive features of your hormones and how to handle them.

## Are my hormones affecting my hair?

Where do we start? First of our hair is a big part of what defines our beauty. The hair on our head is immediately noticeable and the hair where we don't want it is a source of massive anguish. So what's normal?

My practice is in the heart of a beautiful Mediterranean community where wrangling with excess hair is a perennial battle. But I guess because everyone is in the same boat, it doesn't seem to cause as much anguish as thinning hair on top, which is nothing short of a calamity to so many women. There is no strictly defined 'normal' when it comes to hair both on your head and your body.

As far as your facial and body hair goes, lots has to do with your genes, it can be racial and there is a huge range in what is normal. It is completely NORMAL for a woman to have a few hairs on the outer corners of the upper lip, on the chin, around the nipples, on the snail trail between the belly button and pubic area as well as on the tops of the thighs. If your hair growth there is more than just a light growth or if there is coarse hair more widely spread over your face and body, then you have what we call hirsutism or 'excess hair growth'.

You have oestrogen and androgen receptors on your hair follicles. Androgens or male hormones generally make hair grow into the coarser and wirier (like pubic hair), which are called 'terminal hairs' while oestrogen makes your hair softer. Androgens make hair grow in places you don't want, like the body, while androgens make hair on the head thinner and more likely to fall out. Oestrogen stops hair falling out on the head. It also makes the hair softer and smoother. The determination of what hormone receptors grow on which hair follicles on which body parts and in what number is determined largely by your genes. So the hormones coursing through your body may be normal in their levels but there are more receptors on follicles to be activated. Or in cases like polycystic ovarian syndrome, higher androgen levels in the blood mean that male pattern hair growth can push your genes to the extreme.

The normal soft, almost invisible hair that grows on your body is called vellus hair. One of the things androgens do is to convert vellus hairs into terminal hairs. But sometimes, especially after menopause, the vellus hairs start to become more noticeable but are still fine and soft, like 'peach fuzz.' It tends not to worry most women.

# Are my hormones making me hairy?

This is one of the many taboos my patients often don't bring up with me in my practice because women are so embarrassed by it. Women are not supposed to be hairy. Modern women are meant to have thick luscious long hair on our heads and none anywhere else barring perhaps a neat trim landing strip under our tiny g-strings, right? Oh no! That is not the way any of us were designed and so for most of us, we have a lifelong relationship with our wax, local laser hair removal centre, razor or electronic depilator to attempt to defy nature. OK, so that makes you part of the sisterhood. A little leg hair here, some underarm hair there, it's all normal. But what about the hair that grows in unspeakable areas? Around the nipples? On your chin? What's normal? More than you'd think if photos of Miranda Kerr and Candice Swane-poel were your source of information.

Studies in the USA reveal that fully half of all American wom-en regularly remove facial hair and ten per cent of women will remove facial hair two or more times a week. There are women (and you are likely to know quite a few) who have to shave their face once or twice a day because their facial hair grows that quickly. But it's something women never discuss, often not even with their best friends, because they feel so ashamed. The ce-lebrities we see on the pages of our magazines or on TV screens seem to have no hair at all. But hair removal is big business in celeb world, as is making the camera slightly out of focus and retouching still photos.

In all cases of hirsutism, it is testosterone activating the hair follicles that is to blame. But why this is happening can vary in different people. The most common cause is polycystic ovarian syndrome (PCOS) where excess androgens in the blood set the hair follicles on fire. And here is the sad and tragic thing about hirsutism; it's permanent. Once stimulated by your androgens, your hair follicles stay over-active. So for example, a woman might put on some weight and have raised blood androgen lev-els when she is in her late teens or early twenties, and by the time she mentions her problem to the doctor some years later her testosterone levels are normal. However the follicles haven't forgotten their testosterone dance and keep on producing thick, dark androgenic terminal hairs.

All this hair growth starts getting worse in the 40s. There are a couple of reasons for this. First of all, your hair follicles were primed years ago by testosterone, especially if the receptors on your hair follicles are sensitive to testosterone or you had very high circulating levels of testosterone (usually because of PCOS.) In your 40s you start producing less oestrogen. You're still ovulating but you don't get the nice juicy levels you had back in your 30s. So all of a sudden the oestrogen receptors on the hair follicles aren't quite as activated as they used to be but the 'primed' testosterone receptors continue to fire off. In the great hormone battle of the hair on your chin, the testosterone is now winning more often! Voila chin and lip hairs! If you are in your 40s and your tweezer is now your MUST HAVE accessory and you think you're alone – you're so not!

## How to handle your hormones

### BLOOD TESTS

Blood tests. We need to jump through this hoop, especially if you have never been diagnosed with PCOS. These blood tests include androgen levels (including free testosterone, DHEA and sometimes androstenedione) as well as Sex Hormone Binding Globulin (SHBG) and tests for insulin resistance (OGTT with insulin levels). See 'Are My Hormones Making Me Fat?' for more on testing for PCOS and insulin resistance. We are not necessarily looking for whether or not raised androgen levels are causing the hirsutism – they are, we know that for sure. That's not the issue. We are simply trying to find out whether or not you have active PCOS. If you have PCOS, taking specific treatment for PCOS and insulin resistance (mainly metformin plus or minus an anti- androgen pill) will help significantly. Without PCOS or IR metformin would be inappropriate.

### PERMANENT HAIR REMOVAL

Laser and electrolysis are very popular forms of permanent hair removal. With laser, there can be problems with pigmentation if you have either very light or very dark skin. So do a test area first somewhere where it won't matter if you get some pigmentation, like the bikini area. For the back, thighs, bikini area, chest and snail trail it's pretty awesome. Electrolysis allows you to target individual follicles, which is often the case with the upper lip, chin or between the eyebrows. A note about hair on your face; experts say that despite its popularity, tweezing, is the worst way of removing stray hairs from your chin and upper lip. When you tweeze, you often injure the skin. Initially you won't notice anything, but after a while, your skin can become rough and bumpy. If you don't want permanent hair removal or you can't afford it, try a razor or just snipping with scissors or trying bleach so they're not as noticeable. You can also try depilatory creams but they can cause an irritated red rash if you are sensitive to them.

### THE PILL

To even out your hormones and stop your hair follicles being excessively stimulated, you will need to go on the pill unless you are trying to get pregnant. The pill can really help with hair loss, especially if you are using an anti-androgen pill, which has the usual oestrogen but an anti-androgen progesterone formulation such as Cyproterone acetate (in Diane, Brenda or Estelle), drospirenone (in Yasmin or Yaz). I usually favour Cyproterone acetate for hirsutism. These anti-androgen pills cut your circulating testosterone levels by 50 per cent, which is a great start.

### MEDICATIONS

The major anti-androgen medications used for this are spironolactone (such as Spironolactone which is a diuretic drug that inhibits testosterone from activating the receptors) 100 mg a day or Cyproterone acetate (such as Androcur, which again simply deactivates the androgen receptors) for 10 days per month. You start from day five of your menstrual period, and take a 50 mg tablet twice daily for 10 days. It is used in combination with oestrogen (usually the pill). Cyproterone acetate in these doses can give you some weight gain, depression and loss of libido. Studies have shown these medicines work in about 60 per cent of women with hirsutirm but can take six to twelve months to have a good effect. Most of my patients want better results than that.

### EFLORNITHINE HYDROCHLORIDE OR VANIQUA

Eflornithine hydrochloride (or Vaniqua). What a fantastic invention! This cream is used twice a day on clean skin and left on for at least four hours. You don't rub it off. It slows down hair growth on your face (it's not used elsewhere like arms or back) by blocking an enzyme, ornithine decarboxylase in the follicle necessary for hair growth. Lots of my patients see results within four to eight weeks. Sometimes it takes a little longer. It can cause a rash, especially if you have sensitive skin. In that case, you just build up slowly, starting once every second day and over a week or two building up to using it twice a day. It is still incredibly expensive. But not compared to some of the rubbish creams with silly unrealistic anti aging claims you will find at the local cosmetics counter!

# Are my hormones making my hair fall out?

Thinning hair and hair loss are really common complaints in my surgery. Lots of women feel it's a hormone imbalance and like everything else in this book, it probably is PART of the problem.

Female Pattern Hair Loss (FPHL) tends to involve thinning of the hair and shedding especially from the top of the scalp. Doctors who specialise in this area tell me that most women UNDERESTIMATE the extent of their hair loss so when a patient tells me she's worried, I take it seriously.

FPHL has a lot of causes, with your genes taking centre stage. There are both oestrogen and testosterone receptors on your hair follicles but your genes determine how many of each kind. The more oestrogen receptors, the better for your hair and the more testosterone receptors, the worse for hair loss.

In fact any sudden drop in your oestrogen levels can trigger your hair to fall out in masses. The most common one is giving birth where after nine months of glorious, oestrogen fuelled luscious hair, your hair starts falling out all over the place and your shower drain is full of your sheddings! The other times we see accelerated hair loss is in women entering peri-menopause or suddenly stopping their pill. Ironically many women stop the pill because they worry it is the culprit behind their hair loss. In most cases it was simply not doing enough to slow down the hair loss that was going to happen anyway. Once they stop the pill their hair loss really starts accelerating. I promise the pill is not to blame!

All of this can be made worse by a few factors; thyroid disorders. Lack of thyroid hormone can see lots of your hair (not just on your head) dry out, thin and shed easily. So too can iron and zinc deficiency. The other thing that causes it is excess androgens or male hormones from polycystic hormone syndrome. All of these situations will exacerbate the problem that starts with your genetic tendencies. Not everyone with iron deficiency or thyroid problems gets hair loss, but these conditions certainly don't help the situation.

## How to handle your hormones

### BLOOD TESTS

Go to your doctor. By the time you've noticed your thinning hair, you're probably further down the hair loss path than you realise and you need some blood tests. An iron storage (ferritin) level, thyroid hormone tests and blood tests for polycystic ovarian syndrome with androgens and tests for insulin resistance are the first place to start. If you have iron deficiency, thyroid problems or PCOS, head back to the relevant chapters and get them sorted. If blood tests detect zinc deficiency, your doctor will recommend a zinc supplement and retest you after three months with a view to stopping the extra tablets. Zinc overdose is linked to immune system problems so you don't want to be scoffing down masses of zinc without thinking about it.

### MINOXIDIL

This is Rogaine for women. It's a lotion and you rub it onto your scalp every day only where there is obvious hair loss. It takes six to twelve months to reverse the hair loss and you will probably need to stay on it as a maintenance medication long term, but after a year you will no longer need to use it daily. The earlier you get onto it in your hair-loss life, the better, because its ability to reverse the problem has a pretty low ceiling. It is more about halting hair loss so the earlier we get onto the Minoxidil, the better.

### MEDICATION

Again it's the anti-androgen actions of spironolactone (such as Spironolactone, which is a diuretic drug that inhibits testosterone from activating the receptors) at a dose of 100 mg a day or Cyproterone acetate (such as Androcur, which again simply deactivates the androgen receptors) at a dose of 50 mg twice a day for 10

211

days per month that work for hair loss as well. Like the Minoxidil, the earlier you start the better because there's a limit to how much regrowth is achievable and it's more about stopping the further hair loss.

### CONDITION WELL

A leave-in conditioner with silicone can make your hair more manageable and easier to comb so you don't damage it while brushing. That's important because we all lose about 100–200 hairs per day anyway and in your case, each one of these is precious and the fewer lost to wear and tear the better.

### LET YOUR HAIR DRY NATURALLY

We know that wet hair is more easily damaged than dry hair so all that rubbing with a towel is a no-no. If you can avoid blow drying and straightening wet hair, again it will protect the hair from excess wear and tear. Whenever you can, let your hair dry naturally and then style it. Try using a wide-toothed comb and a brush with smooth tips. They rip the hair less.

### GET A GOOD CUT

Get a good cut. At the end of the day, if your hair is really damaged and full of split ends, there is probably not much you can do to repair it. You will have to resort to cutting off all the damaged hair and focus instead on the healthy hair closer to your scalp. Taking good care of that new hair will keep it healthier longer.

# Are my hormones making me break out?

Ok, if you have EVER had a zit, you would have to be living under a rock not to know they're caused by your hormones. All acne is hormonal. Hormones are the starting point of every single zit you ever get. Teenagers start hitting puberty and along with surging levels of testosterone and other androgens, their skin gets oily and they can end up with a 'pizza face'. And for women way past puberty, come pregnancy, or just before a period when your hormones are changing, lots of us get a massive whopper which doesn't make us feel young and lithe, but instead makes us feel ugly and hormonal.

As I said, the culprit is ALWAYS your male hormones. As you already know, we all have male hormones; even us girls, albeit at a tenth of the levels of men. At the very heart of every zit lies these androgens that are converted in the skin to dihydrotestosterone (DHT), which stimulates your oil glands to enlarge and produce the skin's inbuilt moisturizer, sebum. That's a problem. The more sebum your skin makes, the more likely it is that you will have a problem with acne. When the excess sebum together with keratin (dead skin cells) form a blockage in the skin pores, pimples (also known as comedones) can develop. These get infected with bacteria and your immune system mounts an attack on these infected zits. Along with fighting infections, the immune response also brings redness, swelling, and some pain – all of which leads to nasty, red, sore zits.

We know from studies that the earlier the acne starts, the more likely it is to become severe. Teenagers often shrug off their acne and their parents have no idea how devastated they are by the state of their skin. Acne scars can add to the problem. Parents are often nervous about appearing to be critical of their teenager, especially if they're a bit moody anyway. They're afraid if they bring up their teens' acne, they'll damage their self esteem by appearing to call them unattractive. As a parent of a lot of teens (all of them with acne) I get it. But with my doctor's hat on, I see these kids are suffering and would love to be told there is something they can do for their skin. If you are a parent and your teenager has zits, I beg you to chat to them in a loving, supportive non-judgemental way. "I think you're gorgeous, but do you want to go to the doctor to see if we can get something done about those zits?" The sooner you get treatment, the sooner their self esteem gets a boost, and the less chance of scarring.

## How to handle your hormones

GET YOUR BLOOD TESTED

Again it is conditions of excess androgens that we have to look for. If you (or your teen) are found on blood testing to have polycystic ovarian syndrome, it will be important to have specific treatments for PCOS as well as addressing your acne (see Are My Hormones Making Me Fat?')

### IMPROVE YOUR DIET

Regardless of what hormonal imbalances are causing your acne, a diet high in processed foods, as in anything out of a packet, will always make your acne worse. And a diet full of fresh fruit, vegetables, lean meat and fish and dairy will clear up acne. Mind you, many experts think it's the things you're NOT eating that make the most difference to your skin. If you are someone with hormonal issues, whether it's tiredness, your skin, hair loss or weight issues, a good diet is a no-brainer. I know it's hard but it is so important. I suggest you see a good nutritionist for some help. But they have to know what they're talking about. I have seen some seriously bad advice from nutritionists who don't tailor their diets to hormonal problems. Ask your GP for a recommendation to a nutritionist who specialises in this area. I will ONLY refer to two dieticians because I can 100 per cent trust what they tell my patients.

### GET ENOUGH SLEEP

According to the National Sleep Foundation, not getting enough sleep is linked to worse acne in teenagers. One study shows that for every hour of sleep you lose out on, your cortisol levels go up by 14 per cent. We know cortisol makes insulin resistance worse and by now, you all know how that will raise your androgen levels. Like the healthy diet, whether your hormones are causing you to gain weight, feel miserable, break out or feel washed out, you NEED MORE SLEEP!

### GET INTO EXERCISE

We know how exercise sensitises your muscles to insulin, thereby allowing your insulin (and therefore your androgen) levels to fall. Exercise also lowers your cortisol levels, which in turn allows your insulin levels to drop. Just make sure to wash your face after exercise and always wear sunscreen outdoors or risk wrinkles!!! (See following.)

### SKIN CARE FOR ACNE

Acne is not a disease of poor hygiene. It is hormonal and while good skin care will help, it will not solve the problem altogether. Having said all of that, hygiene is a must as a starting point.

Cleansing your skin with a gentle cleanser twice a day is a good way to get rid of the sebum build-up on your skin. You will also need to use a good 'non-comedogenic' moisturiser. Non-comedogenic means non greasy (and so less likely to get stuck in pores and cause pimples.) Avoid toners or things with alcohol in them. Sure they make your skin feel less greasy, but they dry out your skin and can inflame it and make it redder and more sore. Lastly, using Benzoyl peroxide either five or ten per cent can help control the bacteria on your face and can help if the acne is really bad.

### ANTI-ACNE CREAMS

These are the ones on prescription available from your doctor. They're divided roughly into antibiotics that you put on your face (like erythromycin and clindamycin) and creams and potions that help your skin turnover (generate new skin and shed the old stuff) so that it forms healthier skin like Tretinoin (based on vitamin A) and adaptene. All of these work really well if your acne is mild, and you mightn't need anything stronger to control your break outs.

### ANTIBIOTICS

They can be used quite successfully to manage the infections by bacteria called Propionibacterium acnes (*P. acnes*) which is the main bacteria that causes the pussy zits of acne. Unfortunately, over the last 30 years, there has been a massive increase in resistance to antibiotics that we usually use to treat acne. So if you haven't had a response in six to twelve weeks, the likely problem is that it's the wrong antibiotic. See your GP. You can try a different antibiotic, or head for an alternative.

### OTHER MEDICATIONS

Again the anti-androgens, especially spironolactone, can actually be very helpful when added onto the specific anti-PCOS medications (such as metformin) and the anti-androgen pills. Unfortunately dose is key and you can't just have a little homeopathic sniff of spironolactone to get it to work. You will need the full dose of 100 mg a day to get the full anti-acne effect. Plus, it can take a few months to start working.

## METFORMIN

If you have PCOS and high androgen levels, metformin is a fantastic drug that reduces your acne, although you need to give it around four weeks to take effect. In my experience it's underutilised as an anti-acne drug, mainly because doctors still don't test for hormonal problems like PCOS and insulin resistance, just putting your zits down to the usual teenaged hormones. Side effects of metformin can include nausea and tummy gas, but if you start with a low dose and build up slowly, most people can tolerate the side effects.

## THE ANTI-ANDROGEN AND FOURTH GENERATION PILLS

See the Hormone Primer for a recap on how these pills work. Both the pills using either Drospirenone or Cyproterone Acetate as the progestogen block your body's androgens (or male hormones) from activating the androgen receptors in the skin. You will get less oiliness within a fortnight and will start to see fewer pimples within a month. The skin continues to improve over the next six to nine months. Word of warning though: the benefits of these pills are less apparent if you're very over weight, especially from insulin resistance and PCOS. So if you do decide to go on one of these pills, I suggest you head to the chapter Are My Hormones Making Me Fat? and lose some weight either first or at the same time.

## ACCUTANE

The modified vitamin A is your last resort. That's because it has some nasty side effects and you absolutely cannot be pregnant on it because of the birth defects it's been linked to in babies. The side effects are dry lips and eyes, it can make you moody and it has been linked to suicide in some people. It can cause muscle and joint pains, sun sensitivity and higher cholesterol levels. Plus there is a severe but extremely rare side effect of pancreatitis which can be really nasty. Having scared you off, let me tell you that I think many doctors and patients are too afraid of accutane. It's a REALLY effective drug and usually works brilliantly when nothing else has made a dent in the side of the acne. You don't have to use huge doses and you're only on it for as long as it takes to clear up the zits. Many of my patients go on it for six months and don't need to go near it for another three or four years, so long lasting are the results. You should chat to your GP about this if nothing else is working.

## Things that might work

### ZINC CREAMS OR SUPPLEMENTS

There are some pretty reasonable studies now that suggest that using either zinc creams or supplements can be both safe and effective as treatment for acne vulgaris. The reason you won't see it universally promoted though is because other studies have found everything from no effect to negative effects. Some studies have found that low blood levels of zinc are linked to more severe acne, while other studies found absolutely no link at all. So while the jury is out, you can feel free to give it a go, but only for three months. Always get your blood levels of zinc tested before and after using a zinc supplement as excess zinc is linked to a poor immune system function.

### HAVE YOUR MIRENA REMOVED

Studies show anywhere between one in 10 to one in 100 women get worse acne from Mirena. My dermatologist told me that she's had quite a few women in that situation and that pulling out the Mirena cures the problem. If you go back to Chapter one, our hormone primer, you will remember that the Mirena emits around 20 micrograms a day of the first generation progestogen, levonorgestrel. It does have the greatest androgenic effects of all the progestogens, which is probably why it can cause zits. If the Mirena is working for you in every other way, you would probably think twice about that strategy, but it is an option for you.

## Are my hormones making me feel bloated?

They sure can be! There are so many women who talk to me about bloating, I can't believe it. Getting to the bottom of what is causing it can be a real pain.

There are a number of potential candidates:

PMS

As you know, PMS can give you lots of fluid retention. While oestrogen is a water retainer and progesterone is a good diuretic,
you'd think that in the second half of your cycle with progesterone in dominance, you'd get the opposite effect. But progesterone lowers the pressure inside the veins allowing water to escape
into the tissues... If you get bloated towards the end of your cycle
try these hints for a flatter belly:

* Regular exercise has been linked to fewer PMS symptoms,
  including fluid retention.
* Having less salt in your diet can help manage fluid retention. Most of the salt we tend to eat in our diet these
  days comes from an unexpected source; not the salt we
  cook with but the processed foods we eat. Things like soy
  sauce, smoked salmon and deli meats are also packed
  with salt.
* Some of my patients find taking a fluid tablet (diuretic)
  really helpful when they feel bloated during the last part
  of their cycle. It doesn't need to be taken every day, just
  when you feel your tummy blow up. You need a prescription from your doctor.
* Lots of women find either starting a new pill that specifically targets fluid retention (such as one using drospirenone as the progestogen, like Yasmin or Yaz) can be really
  helpful for their PMS related bloating.
* The evidence for other supplements is still patchy. See
  Are My Hormones Making Me Moody? for a full run down
  of PMS supplements.

### An underactive thyroid and constipation

If your thyroid is underactive, one of the major symptoms will be
constipation. As you know, the thyroid hormones speed up the
transition of your food through the gastrointestinal tract so an
underactive thyroid almost always makes you constipated with
the whole transit system winding down to a crawling pace.

So whether it's your hormones, or you're just prone to clogging
up, when it comes to bloating, the number one cause is constipation. So, I thought I'd run through constipation and try to flatten
your belly that way!

Constipation will make you feel very, very, very bloated and distended and will give you buckets of gas. Many women don't realise they're constipated because, contrary to popular myth, constipation doesn't mean you hardly ever make a poop, it means that when the poop comes it comes as a series of pebbles and never gives you the AHA! moment of pure satisfaction that all has been eliminated. What does a healthy poop look like? It's a log! Floating or sinking is irrelevant, but pebbles are a sign of serious poop block.

Fixing it can be tough. I hear women give me the most horrid stories of prune-juice-senna-fibre-supplement cocktails that leave them cramping and stuck at home for hours with massive diarrhoea and back to square one the day after. There are lots of reasons that this treatment regimen is just not the way to go.

## How to handle your constipation

Your large bowel is a very stupid organ. Its job description is simply to remove water from the pre-digested slop that gets delivered to it from the small bowel and then send a formed poop to the outside world. It does this job regardless of whether what is sitting inside is indeed a pre-digested puddle of slop or a cement brick that has been there for several days. Once you have a cement brick sitting inside you, it is pretty hard to move anything. You might get a few pebbles breaking off the brick but will find it much harder to shift the entire traffic jam. Behind it, initially the bowel might cramp up to try and move the jam along, but ultimately it will give up and the bowel's ability to co-ordinate itself into an efficient poop moving tube is gone.

If you pack enough of the usual constipation busters into your system, eventually the bowel will wake up and have a big enough spasm to expel anything. But it's uncomfortable and can give you some nasty diarrhoea to boot. And you will be back to square one in no time.

I cannot stand those fibre or senna-based products. Instead, I use a combination of two products:

   * The first one is a stool softener called macrogol. Its role is to change the cement brick into a sponge that comes out more easily. Macrogol comes in sachets or a tub with

a scooper. Either way you add a certain amount (go by package directions) to any drink and drink it down. You can add it to soup, water, hot tea, juice.... it doesn't matter. The number of sachets and scoops will reflect the number of days since you had a good, ahem, log. So if you've missed one day, you'll have one sachet or scoop per day until you're back on track. If you missed two days, you will have two per day until you're back on track. The maximum is three per day. You can continue to have one every day or every second day as maintenance, especially if you're very prone to constipation and have battled it for years.

* The second product is a liquid paraffin wax. There are quite a few products on the market that contain this greaser. It slides around the outside of your cement brick and lubricates it away from the wall and makes it slide out more easily. You have 30 or 40 ml at night until you've had some lift-off. Like macrogol you can use it as a maintenance tool every night but few people (besides the really frail and immobile elderly) need to go to those lengths.

Both of these products work amazingly well with no cramps and no diarrhoea and perhaps more importantly no rebound constipation once lift off has been achieved.

If you are at this cement brick stage, whatever extra slop is delivered to the large bowel will back up behind the brick making the traffic jam worse. You will end up doubling the size of the cement brick and the problem. For that reason my advice is to stop loading up your large bowel too much and go for a low fibre diet for a few days. I know that's counter intuitive but it actually make sense. We're trying to unblock a drain here. There's no point in making the blockage bigger. So you should have the sort of light diet you would have if you had just recovered from a tummy bug. OK to have:

* Cooked veggies
* Pasta, rice and white bread
* Cooked chicken or fish

Better to avoid
* Raw veggies and salad
* Raw fruit
* High-fibre grains in bread or crackers etc

Once the brick phase has ended and you've had 'lift-off', the light diet is ditched. Instead we're packing in the fibre to try and avoid another cement brick forming. So go for tonnes of fruit, veggies and wholegrains. In every stage drink lots of water to feel brighter and help your bowels along.

If, no wait... WHEN you feel another brick has settled in to hibernate in your large bowel, hop into action quickly. Switch immediately to a light diet and start getting back into macrogol and liquid paraffin ASAP. The sooner you can get the brick out, the less bloated, farty and cranky you will be!

# Are my hormones giving me wrinkles?

I haven't met a woman who embraced her wrinkles, despite all the advice from the feminists. From one woman to another, I hate every line on my face so I get your desire to want to beat them.

Without a doubt, oestrogen is the youth hormone for your face. It puts a little fat under the skin of your face and cheeks. I know you think that sounds crazy, but having a thinner face makes you look older, especially as you hit 40 and beyond. Oestrogen also counteracts the effects of cortisol, which attempts to dismantle the collagen and elastin scaffolding in your skin and make it sag. Oestrogen also keeps your skin looking thicker and healthier.

So with that in mind, let's look at some of the antidotes to the ageing process in your face:

HRT
Nobody would seriously suggest you take HRT for skin ageing alone, but if you go on HRT for the management of your moods, libido, flashes or aches and pains, then we can throw in less ageing on your face and neck for free! It's less clear whether tibolone has the same effect on the face as conventional HRT.

### Stress less

I'm sure you've seen with your own eyes the devastating effects that stressful experiences can have on the face. Have you had a friend who has gone through something dreadful and 'aged ten years'? Chances are it is the higher cortisol levels in her blood that have broken down her collagen and elastin and made her wrinkles deeper. Stress is a youth killer in the face and if nothing else motivates you to manage your stress levels, maybe this will.

### Cut back on the booze

We know that heavy drinkers look older. It is possibly because regular heavy alcohol intake gives you a surge in cortisol (see above). And also we know alcohol makes your tiny blood vessels, the capillaries, leaky, which allows more water into your skin tissue and causes sagging and puffiness.

Safe drinking is 200 ml of wine per day for women. That's two short pours or one heavy pour per day, period!

### Sunscreen

I mean every single day. There are two types of ultraviolet rays from the sun; UVA which is present throughout the day, from early morning until sunset and can penetrate through the glass of your car window. It is the ageing ray. UVB is the one that is harshest in the middle of the day, especially in summer and causes burning. Not ageing. If you think you only need sunscreen in summer at the beach, think again. Your morning drive to work could be ageing your face. Make sure it is a broad spectrum sunscreen that counters both UVA and UVB.

### Moisturise your face (and don't forget your neck!)

Moisturizing traps water in your skin and plumps it up, minimising the appearance of fine lines and wrinkles. Experts tell me that despite the hype and the expensive ingredients, basically moisturisers are moisturisers. Don't look for the fancy-pants ingredients. Instead make sure you are putting enough on.

After washing your face morning and night with water and a soap-free or 'gentle' cleanser, pat your skin dry with your towel instead of rubbing, which can irritate the skin. Then, while your skin is still damp, apply a thin coat of inexpensive moisturiser, such as sorbelene. This will lock the moisture into your skin. You need to moisturize twice a day to keep your skin looking and feeling smoother.

If you are prone to acne, look for an oil-free or 'non-comedo-genic' moisturiser.

### VITAMIN C SERUM (ASCORBIC ACID)

Vitamin C is vital for the production of collagen in your skin plus it is also an antioxidant meaning it neutralises toxic "free radicals", or unstable particles that damage your skin cells.

The skin is the largest organ in the immune system but it is mainly a repellent, keeping chemicals OUT of the body. That's the biggest problem and to get vitamin C to penetrate through the skin it needs to be in an acidic environment firstly and it needs to be in a high concentration, between five and ten per cent ascorbic acid. Unfortunately products that contain that much vitamin C are expensive and it's unlikely that products with low amounts of ascorbic acid have any measurable impact on your skin. The other problem with ascorbic acid in skin-care products is the fact that it is so unstable. When you open a bottle or tube and expose the serum to air it oxidises (like an apple) and its free radical soaking capabilities are pretty well destroyed. What you are left with is a very expensive, fragrant, orangey-smelling cream. In fact if you have ever bought Vitamin C serum, you've probably noticed that the cream around the cap turns brown, which shows that the vitamin C in it has oxidised.

Finally, because it's not a regulated area, the skin care companies don't have to say how much vitamin C is in their product. And even if they did, would you believe them? You can get a therapeutic vitamin C serum made up on prescription from your GP by a compounding chemist.

### VITAMIN A

Like vitamin C, vitamin A is a powerful antioxidant. Plus we know that UV radiation from the sun removes it from our skin making it deficient in some cases. It reverses some ageing as well as sun damage and stimulates collagen production in the skin.

You can put Vitamin A on your skin. It comes in a few forms in cosmetics:

223

* Retinol, which is the natural form of vitamin A has been difficult to get into cosmetics because it is completely unstable and gets broken down by sunlight. But stable preparations are slowly coming onto the market. We don't know exactly how much you need to have in a cream or serum to get a good effect in the skin as this hasn't been properly assessed. But it is probably in very low levels in most over the counter cosmetics because it is frightfully expensive.
* Medical grade Vitamin A or Tretinoin, on the other hand has a constant amount of stable vitamin A and is available on prescription from your GP. It is only approved for acne and using it for ageing skin is using it technically what we call 'off label' (not a government approved use). Having said that, Tretinoin is approved for anti ageing as a twice weekly cream or gel in the USA where it has been found to reduce fine and wrinkles, liver spots and surface roughness. Noticeable improvements take around two to six months.
* Tretinoin makes your skin more sensitive to the sun so wearing sunscreen during the day is even more important. Plus it can cause a red, burning rash at least for a few days but it should all settle down within a few months.

## Vitamin E

There are now some reasonable studies showing that putting vitamin E, especially one of its breakdown products, alpha tocopherol, directly onto your face makes your skin smoother and less wrinkly. Mouse studies have shown it helps protect against skin cancers caused by UV exposure. Again, it's an unregulated area so it's a case of buyer beware when purchasing cosmetics claiming to contain vitamin E.

## Alpha hydroxy acids

Examples of Alpha hydroxy acids include citric, glycolic, malic and tartaric acids. They really do seem to reduce fine lines and wrinkles. Firstly they are great exfoliators, removing the top layer of skin but they also by working deeper in the skin to make it firmer.

Now the problem is that most over the counter products containing alpha hydroxy acids have them in concentrations of between two and ten percent. But studies suggest that to get the anti-ageing benefits, you need closer to 25 percent! And you really need to use them daily for six months to get that sort of excellent result, too. If that's not enough of an issue, at that level, these high-concentration products can irritate the skin, causing nasty redness and burning or itching. You will also be more sensitive to the sun and so wearing a sunscreen every day is a must! We also don't have good data proving that the stronger preparations are safe in pregnancy so if you're thinking of having a baby, put this skin care product away for the time being.

### STEM CELLS

Where do I start? Despite massive celebrity endorsements, there is NO EVIDENCE that PLANT stem cells help human skin. We know from emerging trials that HUMAN stem cells can make enormous gains in wound healing for major injuries such as burns. Watch this space as we are likely to see stem cell treatments for serious skin loss being used regularly within the next few years. But plant stem cells being placed ONTO healthy (if slightly saggy) skin is without scientific back up. Until there is more supportive data, I wouldn't spend money on these products.

### DERMAL FILLERS

Hyaluronic acid is such a popular dermal filler because it occurs naturally within the skin. In your skin, hyaluronic acid acts as a network that transfers essential nutrients from the bloodstream to skin cells. When it is injected under your skin (in a gel formulation), it acts like an inflated cushion and supports the tissues of the face. It's also really hydrating and improves the quality of the skin itself. Like any natural substance, eventually it is broken down and needs to be replaced every six to twelve months. It's not cheap but in the right hands makes the most enormous difference to how young you look.

### BOTULINUM TOXIN (BOTOX)

Botox is the most popular way to minimize frown lines, crows feet and wrinkles on the forehead and neck. Botulinum toxin A and B are both derived from the bacteria that cause botulism. When they're injected into specific areas near wrinkles, the toxin blocks the nerve signals to the muscles, which cause wrinkles to appear by contracting. These days most cosmetic dermatologists and plastic surgeons agree it helps to prevent the formation of new lines and wrinkles as well. It doesn't come cheap and only lasts for three months.

## Procedures to 'resurface' your face

Even if you have wrinkles, having beautiful fresh-looking, well-hydrated skin can make you look years younger. A number of procedures are used to give your skin a makeover.

* Dermabrasion is very popular. Picture your skin being effectively sanded down (planing) the surface layer of your skin with a rapidly rotating brush. This procedure removes the superficial layers of dead skin and a new layer of skin grows in its place. Don't plan a big night out after a session of dermabrasion. You will probably have a pretty red face and you won't want to have make up on it, especially if it feels a little tender. Use more sunscreen than usual in the weeks after because you will burn more easily with this new skin on your face.
* Microdermabrasion, is a lighter, somewhat gentler version of dermabrasion with less skin cells removed. It tends to last a shorter time and is often done by beauticians in salons. Despite the 'light' version, a 2009 study published in the *Archives of Dermatology* not only showed that microdermabrasion does indeed decrease the appearance of fine lines and wrinkles but that it actually made the skin make more collagen (the skin's own natural scaffolding that tends to sag a bit as we age). After microdermabrasion the redness will only last a couple of hours.
* Chemical peels use chemicals to remove the uneven top layer of skin to get a smoother surface for the skin. Generally phenol, trichloroacetic acid and alphahydroxy acids are used in different combinations. The hydroxyacids include glycolic acid, lactic acid, salicylic acid and maleic acid. The chemicals are applied to your face, allowed to

sit (the time varies depending on the specific chemicals used and whether you are doing a light, medium or deep chemical peel). Then they are washed off using water or saline. Deep peels make your face look HORRIBLE (and feel painful for that matter) for a couple of days. Whereas a light peel will just give some mild stinging immediately but you leave the surgery feeling and looking great. The strength of the peel depends on the degree of ageing and what you are trying to achieve with the procedure.

# Are my hormones making me look blotchy?

More than 90 per cent of people who get pigmentation blotches on the face, called melasma are women. While it is definitely brought on by exposure to the sun, it typically happens with hormonal changes, like going on the pill or HRT or getting pregnant. We don't understand how the hormones interact with the pigment-producing cells in the skin but stopping the HRT or the pill or giving birth usually sort out hormonal melasma quick smart.

Melasma is definitely genetic – it runs in families. And it tends to be more common in people who are darker skinned such as Mediterranean and Middle Eastern women.

## How to handle your melasma

### HYDROQUINONE

This ingredient in skin creams actually removes pigment from the skin directly. It can start working after only two weeks of treatment, though worse melasma might take a little longer. You can find hydroquinone-containing products in over-the-counter cosmetics. The dose is either two per cent or even less. You can get a more effective four-per cent hydroquinone preparation on prescription from your doctor.

It is often given with medical grade Tretinoin and sometimes a mild hydrocortisone is added. This is usually compounded into a single cream with a custom prescription from your doctor.

### Sun avoidance

If sunshine is making you blotchy, you have to wear a hat, apply 30 plus sunscreen and avoid sunlight to the face as much as possible.

### Procedures for melasma

If a cream and sun avoidance don't clear up your melasma, you can try a procedure. A high-quality chemical peel (such as glycolic acid), microdermabrasion and dermabrasion have all been used by dermatologists successfully. They should be done by a cosmetic physician.

# Are my hormones making me spotty?

Age spots, or solar lentigines are also known as 'liver spots'. They are flat grey, brown or black spots. They're most commonly found on the face, hands, shoulders and arms, which tend to be the areas that cop most sun exposure over a lifetime. They become much more common after you hit 40, but younger people can get them as well. And no, unlike melasma, hormones do not play any part whatsoever. They're all about age. I thought I'd cover them here because we have dealt with an ageing face.

There was a study recently that found it is the pigmentation spots on your skin that make you look older than your wrinkles.

## How to handle your spots

### Sunscreen

These spots are caused by sun damage. Check out my UVA and UVA tips above and grab yourself some sunscreen and start being diligent to prevent more liver spots cropping up. Every day, whether you're off to the beach or not, it's never too late!

### Bleaching creams

Prescription bleaching creams (like hydroquinone – see above) can help reduce the amount of pigment to make them less noticeable. Sometimes they're given with prescription strength retinoids (Tretinoin) and a mild steroid or used alone (as for melasma). This can make them gradually fade over several months.

### LASER

Laser therapies can destroy melanin or pigment producing cells without damaging the skin's surface. Treatments with a laser typically require several sessions. After treatment, age spots fade gradually over several weeks or months. The Q switch laser is especially good for this problem.

### DERMABRASION

Dermabrasion can be fantastic for removing liver spots. The same dermabrasion you would get for general aging, fine lines and wrinkles is used.

### CHEMICAL PEEL

Chemical peels can be really effective for removing liver spots as well as making fine lines and wrinkles much less noticeable. If you go for a deep peel expect to stay inside slathered with some petroleum jelly for two days before emerging back into the real world. The new skin is very sensitive to the sun so you need to diligently apply 30 plus sunscreen every day.

# Are my hormones giving me cellulite?

Fat is basically anchored down onto the body by a kind of mesh of connective tissue. In men, this mesh network is reasonably strong, while in women, it is weaker and tends to distort more easily allowing the fat beneath to bulge out into the overlying skin, creating a dimpling effect.

All doctors agree that hormones play a role in the development of cellulite because of the difference in the structure of that connective tissue meshwork. It mainly happens to women and in the areas that oestrogen orders our bodies to place fat such as the thighs, hips and butt. But what role hormones play and which hormones are to blame remains unknown.

## How to handle your cellulite

Ladies I am not a fountain of good news here.

Losing weight is the first piece of advice. Weight loss has been shown to improve the appearance of cellulite. But girls we all know that weight loss only does so much.

Therapies have focused on breaking down fat by using substances such as caffeine, laser and even infra-red light. Not much to report yet, but watch this space. Doctors are really optimistic, especially about carefully targeted laser beams.

A number of anti-cellulite machines have come to the market in recent years, but doctors are loath to endorse them. It seems that at best the ones done in the rooms of clinicians provide a 20 to 25 per cent improvement for an enormous outlay of money and that they need to be done continuously. The DIY ones that you buy at home or enrol for at a non-medical gym seem to have even less impressive results.

Rubbing a 0.3 per cent retinol cream onto cellulite-ridden skin twice a day has been shown to improve the appearance of cellulite after six months. Not sure whether you need to continue that indefinitely. Plus that's a pretty strong mixture. It isn't available commercially and needs to be specially made for you by a compounding chemist.

## What won't work

### COFFEE

Rubbing coffee granules on your butt. While caffeine itself may have an effect on cellulite, rubbing coffee granules onto your skin is pointless, since the caffeine can't escape the granules to penetrate the skin.

### LIPOSUCTION

Oh it will remove fat alright. But it won't get rid of cellulite. In fact, it can make cellulite worse by making deeper depressions in the skin.

### CELLULITE CREAMS

I can't believe some of the labels on anti-cellulite creams are legal. None of the claims are evidence-based. They're SO expensive and I've never met anybody who said they work.

# The last word

Thanks for sticking with me. I hope by now you have a good understanding of the hormones in your life, how they're affecting your mind, body and spirit and how you can take back control. Best of luck with everything.

Ginni xxxxx

Also by Dr Ginni Mansberg

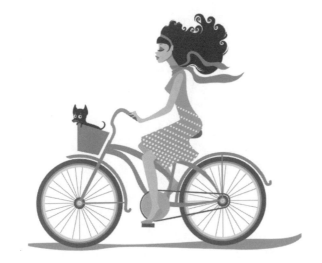

*How to Get Your Mojo Back*

Every Woman's Guide to Health and Happiness

DR GINNI MANSBERG

ISBN 9781741109245

Also available as an ebook.

First published in 2013 by New Holland Publishers Pty Ltd
London • Sydney • Cape Town • Auckland

Garfield House 86–88 Edgware Road London W2 2EA United Kingdom
1/66 Gibbes Street Chatswood NSW 2067 Australia
Wembley Square First Floor Solan Road Gardens Cape Town 8001 South Africa
218 Lake Road Northcote Auckland New Zealand

www.newhollandpublishers.com

A record of this book is held at the British Library or the National Library of
Australia.

ISBN 9 781 74257 231 4

Managing Director: Fiona Schultz
Publishing Manager: Lliane Clarke
Editor: Simona Hill
Proofreader: Catherine Etteridge
Production Director: Olga Dementiev
Cover Design: Kimberley Pearce
Printer: Ligare Pty Ltd

10 9 8 7 6 5 4 3 2 1

Keep up with New Holland Publishers on Facebook

www.facebook.com/NewHollandPublishers